CONTRIBUTIONS
TO THE ANALYSIS
OF THE SENSATIONS

CONTRIBUTIONS
TO THE ANALYSIS
OF THE SENSATIONS

ERNST MACH

Translated by C. M. Williams

with thirty-seven cuts

THE OPEN COURT PUBLISHING COMPANY
La Salle, Illinois

PREFACE TO THE ENGLISH EDITION.

FOR the preparation of the present excellent translation of my *Beiträge zur Analyse der Empfindungen* I am under profound obligations to The Open Court Publishing Company Not a little of the progress of psychology is owing to the strenuous efforts which the promoters of the science have made to find the main explanation of its problems in the principle of association and these investigations have received a fresh impulse from the results of neural anatomy and neural physiology. I am of opinion however, that the idea advanced in the present work, agreeably to which as many physico-chemical neural processes are to be assumed as there are distinguishable qualities of sensation, is also possessed of heuristic value, and that there is reasonable hope that at some future time it, too, will receive elucidation from the side of physiological chemistry. Admittedly, this idea, which is but a consistent, monistic conception of Müller's principle of the specific energies, is not in accord with prevailing notions. By the example and influence of a great authority it has become the custum to relegate the explanation of *different qualities* of sensation to unknown domains, and to regard all neural processes as absolutely alike qualitatively and only quantitatively different. I had occasion as early as 1863 (*Vorlesungen über Psychophysik*, Vienna, Sommer, p. 33) to point out how little such a conception is calculated to lead to a profounder knowledge of our sensations, and how little justifiable it is, even from a physical point of view, to regard all electric neural currents as physical processes qualitatively the same in kind. One has only to think of a current through copper, through sulphate of copper, or through acidulated water. A few inquirers only, like Hering, still uphold Müller's doctrine in its original signification, and under these circumstances the opportunity of presenting my thoughts to a new public is doubly valuable.

E. MACH.

VIENNA, September, 1896.

ORIGINAL PREFACE.

THE frequent excursions which I have made into this province
have all sprung from the profound conviction that the foun-
dations of science as a whole, and of physics in particular, await
their next greatest elucidations from the side of biology, and especially from the analysis of the sensations.

I am aware, of course, that I can contribute but little to the
attainment of this end. The very fact that my investigations have
been carried on, not in the way of a profession, but only at odd
moments, and frequently only after long interruptions, must de-
tract considerably from the value of my scattered publications, or
perhaps even lay me open to the secret charge of desultoriness
So much the more, therefore, am I under especial obligations to
those investigators, such as E. Hering, V. Hensen, W. Preyer
and others, who have directed attention either to the matter of my
writings or to their methodological outcome.

The present compendious and supplementary presentation of
my views, perhaps, will place my attitude in a somewhat more
favorable light, for it will be seen that in all cases I have had in
mind the *same problem*, no matter how varied or numerous were
the single facts investigated. Although I can lay no claim whatever to the title of physiologist, and still less to that of philosopher,
yet I venture to hope that the work thus undertaken, purely from
a strong desire for self-enlightenment, by a physicist unconstrained
by the conventional barriers of the specialist, may not be entirely

without value for others also, even though I may not be every-where in the right.

My natural bent for the study of these questions received its strongest stimulus from Fechner's *Elemente der Psychophysik* (Leipsic, 1860), but my greatest assistance was derived from Hering's solution of the two problems referred to in the footnote of page 35 and in the text of page 81.

To readers who, for any reason, desire to avoid more general discussions, I recommend the omission of the first and last chapters. For me, however, the conception of the whole and the conception of the parts are so intimately related that I should scarcely be able to separate them.

THE AUTHOR.

PRAGUE, November, 1885.

TRANSLATOR'S NOTE.

THE MATTER contained in a book is by no means propor-
tioned to its size. If this were so, the following treatise,
rich as it is in suggestions bearing on some of the fundamental
problems of scientific and philosophical theory, must be a bulky
one. The author has not, however, entered into any detailed application of the conclusions drawn from his observations and experiments, but has contented himself with a succinct exposition of
those conclusions, leaving to the reader the very pleasurable task
of following out the many trains of thought opened up by them
The German edition of the book has been the subject of great interest and discussion. To the English text the author has added
considerable new matter in the notes on pages 4, 20, 21, 26, 39,
40, 56, 78, 82–83, 115, and in the two Appendices.

The manuscript and proofs of this edition have had the advantage of revisal by Mr. T. J. McCormack, of La Salle, Illinois
translator of the author's *Science of Mechanics*, who also independently rendered the "Introductory Remarks" and Appendix I.
—matter which originally appeared in *The Monist*.

C. M. WILLIAMS.

BOSTON, December, 1896.

CONTENTS.

CONTRIBUTIONS
TO THE ANALYSIS
OF THE SENSATIONS

INTRODUCTORY REMARKS.

ANTIMETAPHYSICAL.

I.

THE splendid success achieved by physical science in modern times, a success which is not restricted to its own sphere but embraces that of other sciences which employ its help, has brought it about that physical ways of thinking and physical modes of procedure enjoy on all hands unwonted prominence, and that the greatest expectations are associated with their employment. In keeping with this drift of modern inquiry, the physiology of the senses, gradually leaving the paths which were opened by men like Goethe, Schopenhauer, and others, but with particular success by Johannes Müller, has also assumed an almost exclusively physical character. This tendency must appear to us as not exactly the proper one, when we reflect that physics despite its considerable development nevertheless constitutes but a portion of a *larger* collective body of knowledge, and that it is unable, with its limited intellectual implements, created for limited and special purposes, to exhaust all the subject-matter

of science.   Without renouncing the support of physics, it is possible for the physiology of the senses, not
only to pursue its own course of development, but also
to afford to physical science itself powerful assistance ;
a point which the following simple considerations will
serve to illustrate.

2.

Colors, sounds, temperatures, pressures, spaces,
times, and so forth, are connected with one another in
manifold ways; and with them are associated moods of
mind, feelings, and volitions.   Out of this fabric, that
which is relatively more fixed and permanent stands
prominently forth, engraves itself in the memory, and
expresses itself in language.   Relatively greater permanency exhibit, first, certain *complexes* of colors,
sounds, pressures, and so forth, connected in time and
space, which therefore receive special names, and are
designated *bodies*.   Absolutely permanent such complexes are not.

My table is now brightly, now dimly lighted.   Its
temperature varies.   It may receive an ink stain.   One
of its legs may be broken.   It may be repaired, polished,
and replaced part for part.   But for me, amid all its
changes, it remains the table at which I daily write.

My friend may put on a different coat.   His countenance may assume a serious or a cheerful expression.
His complexion, under the effects of light or emotion,
may change.   His shape may be altered by motion,

or be definitely changed. Yet the number of the permanent features presented, compared with the number of the gradual alterations, is always so great, that the latter may be overlooked. It is the same friend with whom I take my daily walk.

My coat may receive a stain, a tear. My very manner of expression shows that we are concerned here with a sum-total of permanency, to which the new element is added and from which that which is lacking is subsequently taken away.

Our greater intimacy with this sum-total of permanency, and its preponderance as contrasted with the changeable, impel us to the partly instinctive, partly voluntary and conscious economy of mental representation and designation, as expressed in ordinary thought and speech. That which is perceptually represented in a single image receives *a single* designation, *a single* name.

As relatively permanent, is exhibited, further, that complex of memories, moods, and feelings, joined to a particular body (the human body), which is denominated the "I" or "Ego." I may be engaged upon this or that subject, I may be quiet or animated, excited or ill-humored. Yet, pathological cases apart, enough durable features remain to identify the ego. Of course, the ego also is only of relative permanency.[1]

---

[1]The apparent permanency of the ego consists chiefly in the fact of its *continuity* and in the slowness of its changes. The many thoughts and plans of yesterday that are continued to-day, and of which our environment in waking hours incessantly reminds us (wherefore in dreams the ego can be very in-

After a first survey has been obtained, by the formation of the substance-concepts "body" and "ego" (matter and soul), the will is impelled to a more exact examination of the *changes* that take place in these relatively permanent existences. The changeable features of bodies and of the ego, in fact, are exactly what moves the will to this examination. Here the component parts of the complex are first exhibited as its

distinct, doubled, or entirely wanting), and the little habits that are unconsciously and involuntarily kept up for long periods of time, constitute the groundwork of the ego. There can hardly be greater differences in the egos of different people, than occur in the course of years in *one* person. When I recall to-day my early youth, I should take the boy that I then was, with the exception of a few individual features, for a different person, did not the chain of memories that make up my personality lie actually before me. Many an article that I myself penned twenty years ago impresses me now as something quite foreign to myself. The very gradual character of the changes of the body also contributes to the stability of the ego, but in a much less degree than people imagine. Such things are much less analysed and noticed than the intellectual and the moral ego. Personally, people know themselves very poorly.

Once, when a young man, I espied in the street the profile of a face that was very displeasing and repulsive to me. I was not a little taken aback when a moment afterwards I found that it was my own, which, in passing by a place where mirrors were sold, I had perceived reflected from two mirrors that were inclined at the proper angle to each other.

Not long ago, after a trying railway journey by night, and much fatigued, I got into an omnibus, just as another gentleman appeared at the other end. "What degenerate pedagogue is that, that has just entered," thought I. It was myself: opposite me hung a large mirror. The physiognomy of my class, accordingly, was better known to me than my own.

The ego is as little absolutely permanent as are bodies. That which we so much dread in death, the annihilation of our permanency, actually occurs in life in abundant measure. That which is most valued by us, remains preserved in countless copies, or, in cases of exceptional excellence, is even preserved of itself. In the best human being, however, there are individual traits, the loss of which neither he himself nor others need regret. Indeed, at times, death, viewed as a liberation from individuality, may even become a pleasant thought. [When I wrote these lines, Ribot's admirable little book, *The Diseases of Personality*, second edition, Paris, 1888, Chicago, 1895, was unknown to me. Ribot ascribes the principal rôle in preserving the continuity of the ego to the general sensibility. Generally, I am in perfect accord with his views.—Mach, 1895.]

properties. A fruit is sweet; but it can also be bitter. Also, other fruits may be sweet. The red color we are seeking is found in many bodies. The neighborhood of some bodies is pleasant ; that of others, unpleasant. Thus, gradually, different complexes are found to be made up of common elements. The visible, the audible, the tangible, are separated from bodies. The visible is analysed into colors and into form. In the manifoldness of the colors, again, though here fewer in number, other component parts are discerned— such as the primary colors, and so forth. The complexes are disintegrated into *elements*.

3.

The useful habit of designating such relatively permanent compounds by *single* names, and of apprehending them by *single* thoughts, without going to the trouble each time of an analysis of their component parts, is apt to come into strange conflict with the tendency to isolate the component parts. The vague image which we have of a given permanent complex, being an image which does not perceptibly change when one or another of the component parts is taken away, gradually establishes itself as something which exists *by itself*. Inasmuch as it is possible to take away *singly* every constituent part without destroying the capacity of the image to *stand for* the totality and of being recognised again, it is imagined that it is possible to subtract *all* the parts and to have something still remaining. Thus arises the monstrous notion of a *thing in itself*, unknowable and different from its "phenomenal" existence.

Thing, body, matter, are nothing apart from their complexes of colors, sounds, and so forth—nothing apart from their so-called attributes. That Protean, supposititious problem, which springs up so much in philosophy, of a *single* thing with *many* attributes, arises wholly from a mistaking of the fact, that summary comprehension and precise analysis, although both are provisionally justifiable and for many purposes profitable, cannot and must not be carried on *simultaneously*. A body is one and unchangeable only so long as it is unnecessary to consider its details. Thus both the earth and a billiard-ball are spheres, if the purpose in hand permits our neglecting deviations from the spherical form, and great precision is not necessary. But when we are obliged to carry on investigations in orography or microscopy, both bodies cease to be spheres.

4.

Man possesses, in its highest form, the power of consciously and arbitrarily determining his point of view. He can at one time disregard the most salient features of an object, and immediately thereafter give attention to its smallest details; now consider a stationary current, without a thought of its contents, and then measure the width of a Fraunhofer line in the spectrum; he can rise at will to the most general abstractions or bury himself in the minutest particulars. The animal possesses this capacity in a far less degree. It does not assume a point of view, but is usually forced to it. The babe who does not know its father with his hat on, the dog that is perplexed at the new coat of its master, have both succumbed in this conflict of points of view. Who has not been worsted in similar plights? Even the man of philosophy at times succumbs, as the grotesque problem, above referred to, shows.

In this last case, the circumstances appear to furnish a real ground of justification. Colors, sounds, and the odors of bodies are evanescent. But the tangible part, as a sort of constant, durable nucleus, not readily susceptible of annihilation, remains behind; appearing as the vehicle of the more fugitive properties annexed to it. Habit, thus, keeps our thought firmly attached to this central nucleus, even where the knowledge exists that seeing, hearing, smelling, and *touching* are intimately akin in character. A further consideration is, that owing to the singularly extensive development of mechanical physics a kind of *higher reality* is ascribed to space and time than to colors, sounds, and odors; agreeably to which, the temporal and spatial *links* of colors, sounds, and odors appear to be *more real* than the colors, sounds, and odors themselves. The physiology of the senses, however, demonstrates, that spaces and times may just as appropriately be called sensations as colors and sounds.

5.

The ego, and the relation of bodies to the ego, give rise to similar pseudo-problems, the character of which may be briefly indicated as follows :

Let those complexes of colors, sounds, and so forth, commonly called bodies, be designated, for the sake of simplicity, by $ABC\ldots$; the complex, known as our own body, which constitutes a part of the former, may be called $KLM\ldots$; the complex composed of volitions, memory-images, and the rest, we shall represent by $\alpha\beta\gamma\ldots$ Usually, now, the complex $\alpha\beta\gamma\ldots$ $KLM\ldots$, as making up the ego, is opposed to the complex $ABC\ldots$, as making up the world of substance; sometimes, also, $\alpha\beta\gamma\ldots$ is viewed as ego, and $KLM\ldots ABC\ldots$ as world of substance. Now, at first blush, $ABC\ldots$ appears independent of the ego, and opposed to it as a separate existence. But this independence is only relative, and gives way upon closer inspection.   Much, it is true, may change in the complex $\alpha\beta\gamma\ldots$ without a perceptible change being induced in $ABC\ldots$; and *vice versa*. But many changes in $\alpha\beta\gamma\ldots$ do pass, by way of changes in $KLM\ldots$, to $ABC\ldots$; and *vice versa*. (As, for example, when powerful ideas burst forth into acts, or our environment induces noticeable changes in our body.) At the same time the group $KLM\ldots$ appears to be more intimately connected with $\alpha \beta \gamma \ldots$ and with $A B C \ldots$, than the latter do with one another; relations which find their expression in common thought and speech.

Precisely viewed, however, it appears that the group $A B C \ldots$ is *always* codetermined by $K L M$. A cube of wood when seen close at hand, looks large; when seen at a distance, small; it looks different with the right eye from what it does with the left; sometimes it appears double; with closed eyes it is invisible. The properties of the same body, therefore, appear modified by our own body; they appear conditioned by it. But where, now, is that *same* body, which to the appearance is so *different* ? All that can be said is, that with different $K L M$ different $A B C \ldots$ are associated.[1]

We see an object having a point S. If we touch S, that is, bring it into connexion with our body, we receive a prick. We can see S, without feeling the prick. But as soon as we feel the prick we find S. The visible point, therefore, is a *permanent fact* or *nu-*

[1] A long time ago (in the *Vierteljahrsschrift für Psychiatrie*, Leipsic and Neuwied, 1868, art. "Ueber die Abhängigkeit der Netzhautstellen von einander," I enunciated this thought as follows: The expression "sense-illusion" proves that we are not yet fully conscious, or at least have not yet deemed it necessary to incorporate the fact into our ordinary language, *that the senses represent things neither wrongly nor correctly.* All that can be truly said of the sense-organs is, that, *under different circumstances they produce different sensations and perceptions.* As these "circumstances," now, are extremely manifold in character, being partly external (inherent in the objects), partly internal (inherent in the sensory organs), and partly interior (having their seat in the central organs), it would naturally seem, especially when attention is paid only to external circumstances, as if the organs acted differently under the same conditions. And it is customary to call the unusual effects, deceptions or illusions.

cleus, to which the prick is annexed, according to circumstances, as something accidental. From the frequency of such occurrences we ultimately accustom ourselves to regard *all* properties of bodies as "effects" proceeding from permanent nuclei and conveyed to the ego through the medium of the body ; which effects we call *sensations*. By this operation, however, our imagined nuclei are deprived of their entire sensory contents, and converted into mere mental symbols. The assertion, then, is correct that the world consists only of our sensations. In which case we have knowledge *only* of sensations, and the assumption of the nuclei referred to, or of a reciprocal action between them, from which sensations proceed, turns out to be quite idle and superfluous. Such a view can only suit with a half-hearted realism or a half-hearted philosophical criticism.

6.

Ordinarily the complex $\alpha \beta \gamma \ldots KLM \ldots$ is contrasted as ego with the complex ABC. Those elements only of $ABC \ldots$ that more strongly alter $\alpha \beta \gamma \ldots$, as a prick, a pain, are wont to be comprised in the ego. Afterwards, however, through observations of the kind just referred to, it appears that the right to annex $ABC \ldots$ to the ego nowhere ceases. In conformity with this view the ego can be so extended as ultimately to embrace the entire world.[1] The ego is not sharply

[1] When I say that the table, the tree, and so forth, are my sensations, the statement, as contrasted with the mode of representation of the ordinary man,

marked off, its limits are very indefinite and arbitrarily displaceable.   Only by failing to observe this fact, and by unconsciously narrowing those limits, while at the same time we enlarge them, arise, in the conflict of points of view, the metaphysical difficulties met with in this connexion.

As soon as we have perceived that the supposed unities "body" and "ego" are only makeshifts, designed for provisional survey and for certain practical ends (so that we may take hold of bodies, protect *ourselves* against pain, and so forth), we find ourselves obliged, in many profound scientific investigations, to abandon them as insufficient and inappropriate.   The antithesis of ego and world, sensation (phenomenon) and thing, then vanishes, and we have simply to deal with the *connexion* of the *elements* $\alpha \beta \gamma \ldots A B C \ldots K L M \ldots$, of which this antithesis was only a partially appropriate and imperfect expression.   This connexion is nothing more nor less than the combination of the above-mentioned elements with other similar elements (time and space).   Science has simply to *accept* this connexion, and to set itself aright (get its bearings) in the intellectual environment which is thereby furnished, without attempting to explain its existence.

---

involves a real extension of my ego.   On the emotional side also such extensions occur, as in the case of the virtuoso, who possesses as perfect a mastery of his instrument as he does of his own body; or in the case of the skilful orator, on whom the eyes of the audience are all converged, and who is controlling the thoughts of all; or in that of the able politician who is deftly guiding his party; and so on.   In conditions of depression, on the other hand such as nervous people often endure, the ego contracts and shrinks.   A wall seems to separate it from the world.

On a superficial examination the complex $\alpha\beta\gamma\ldots$ appears to be made up of much more evanescent elements than $A B C\ldots$ and $K L M\ldots$ in which last the elements seem to be connected with greater *stability* and *in a more permanent manner* (being joined to solid nuclei as it were).   Although on closer inspection the elements of all complexes prove to be *homogeneous*, yet in spite of the knowledge of this fact, the early notion of an antithesis of body and spirit easily regains the ascendancy in the mind. The philosophical spiritualist is often sensible of the difficulty of imparting the needed solidity to his mind-created world of bodies ; the materialist is at a loss when required to endow the world of matter with sensation. The *monistic* point of view, which artificial reflexion has evolved, is easily clouded by our older and more powerful instinctive notions.

7.

The difficulty referred to is particularly felt in the following case.   In the complex $A B C\ldots$, which we have called the world of matter, we find as parts, not only our own body $K L M\ldots$, but also the bodies of other persons (or animals) $K'L'M'\ldots$, $K''L''M''\ldots$, to which, by analogy, we imagine other $\alpha'\beta'\gamma'\ldots$, $\alpha''\beta''\gamma''\ldots$, annexed, similar to $\alpha\beta\gamma\ldots$ So long as we deal with $K'L'M'\ldots$, we find ourselves in a thoroughly familiar province at every point sensorially accessible to us. When, however, we inquire after the sensations or feelings appurtenant to the body

K'L'M'..., we no longer find the elements we seek in the province of sense: *we add them in thought*. Not only is the domain which we now enter far less familiar to us, but the transition into it is also relatively unsafe. We have the feeling as if we were plunging into an abyss.[1] Persons who adopt this method only, will never thoroughly rid themselves of this sense of insecurity, which is a frequent source of illusive problems.

But we are not restricted to this course. Let us consider, first, the reciprocal relations of the elements of the complex *A B C*..., without regarding *K L M*... (our body). All physical investigations are of this sort. A white bullet falls upon a bell; a sound is heard. The bullet turns yellow before a sodium lamp, red before a lithium lamp. Here the elements (*ABC*...) appear to be connected only *with one another* and to be independent of our body (*K L M*...). But if we take santonine, the bullet again turns yellow. If we press one eye to the side, we see two bullets. If we close our eyes entirely, we see none at all. If we sever the

[1] When I first came to Vienna from the country, as a boy of four or five years, and was taken by my father upon the walls of the city's fortifications, I was very much surprised to see people below in the moat, and could not understand how, from my point of view, they could have got there; for the thought of another way of descent never occurred to me. I remarked the same astonishment, once afterwards in life, in the case of a three-year-old boy of my own, while walking on the walls of Prague. I recall this feeling every time I occupy myself with the reflexion of the text, and I frankly confess that this accidental experience of mine helped to confirm my opinion upon this point, which I have now long held. The habit of pursuing the same methods in material and psychical questions tends greatly to confuse our field of survey. A child, on the piercing of the wall of a house in which it has long dwelt, may experience a veritable enlargement of its world-view, and in the same manner a slight scientific hint may often afford great enlightenment.

auditory nerve, no sound is heard. The elements
$A B C \ldots$, therefore, are not only connected among
one another, but also with $K L M$. To this extent,
and to this extent *only*, do we call $A B C \ldots$ *sensations*,
and regard $A B C$ as belonging to the ego. In this way,
accordingly, we do not find the gap between bodies
and sensations above described, between what is without and what is within, between the material world
and the spiritual world.[1] All elements $A B C \ldots$,
$K L M \ldots$ constitute a *single* coherent mass only, in
which, when any one element is disturbed, *all* is put
in motion; except that a disturbance in $K L M \ldots$ has
a more extensive and profound action than in $A B C$.
A magnet in our neighborhood disturbs the particles
of iron near it; a falling boulder shakes the earth;
but the severing of a nerve sets in motion the *whole*
system of elements.[2]

8.

That traditional gulf between physical and psychological research, accordingly, exists only for the habit-
ual stereotyped method of observation.   A color is a
physical object so long as we consider its dependence
upon its luminous source, upon other colors, upon
heat, upon space, and so forth. Regarding, however, its
dependence upon the retina (the elements $K L M \ldots$),

[1] Compare my *Grundlinien der Lehre von den Bewegungsempfindungen*
Leipsic: Engelmann, 1875, p. 54.

[2] Quite involuntarily does this relation of things suggest the picture of a
viscous mass, at certain places (as in the ego) more firmly coherent than in
others.   I have often made use of this simile in lectures.

it becomes a psychological object, a sensation. Not the subject, but the direction of our investigation, is different in the two domains.

Both in reasoning from the observation of the bodies of other men or animals, to the sensations which they possess, as well as in investigating the influence of our own body upon our own sensations, we must complete observed facts by analogy. This is accomplished with much greater readiness and certainty, when it relates, say, only to nervous processes, which cannot be fully observed in our own bodies—that is, when it is carried out in the more familiar physical domain—than when it is made in connexion with psychical processes. Otherwise there is no essential difference.

9.

The considerations advanced will gain in strength and vividness by a concrete example. Thus, I lie upon my sofa. If I close my right eye, the picture represented in the accompanying cut is presented to my left eye. In a frame formed by the ridge of my eyebrow, by my nose, and by my moustache, appears a part of my body, so far as visible, with its environment.[1] *My* body differs from other human bodies— beyond the fact that every intense motor idea is immediately expressed by a movement of it, and that its

---

[1] A discussion of the binocular field of vision, with its peculiar stereoscopic features, is omitted here, for although familiar to all, it is not as easy to describe, and cannot be represented by a single plane drawing.

being touched determines more striking changes than contact with other bodies—by the circumstance, that it is only partly seen, and, especially, is seen without

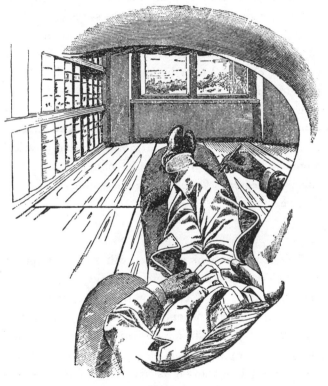

Fig. 1.

a head.   If I observe an element A within my field of vision, and investigate its connexion with another element B within the same field, I step out of the domain of physics into that of physiology or psychology, provided *B*, to use the apposite expression of a friend[1] of mine made upon seeing this drawing, passes through my skin. Reflexions like that for the field of vision may be made with regard to the province of touch and the perceptual domains of the other senses.

10.

Reference has already been made to the different character of the groups of elements designated by *A B C* . . . and *α β γ*. As a matter of fact, when we *see* a green tree before us, or *remember* a green tree, that is, represent a green tree to ourselves, we are perfectly aware of the difference of the two cases. The represented tree has a much less determinate, a much more changeable form ; its green is much paler and more evanescent ; and, what is of especial note, it is plainly situate in a *different* domain. A movement that we *propose* to execute is never more than a represented movement, and appears in a different sphere from that of the executed movement, which always takes place when the image is vivid enough. The statement that the elements *A* and *α* appear in different spheres, means, if we go to the bottom of it, simply this, that these elements are united with different other elements. Thus far, therefore, the fundamental constituents of *A B C* . . ., *α β γ* . . . would seem to be *the same* (colors, sounds, spaces, times, motor sensations

[1] J. Popper of Vienna.

. . .), and only the character of their connexion different.

Ordinarily pleasure and pain are regarded as different from sensations. Yet not only tactile sensations, but all other kinds of sensations, may pass gradually into pleasure and pain. Pleasure and pain also may be justly termed sensations. Only they are not so well analysed and so familiar as the common sensations. In fact, sensations of pleasure and pain, however faint they may be, really make up the contents of all so-called emotions. Thus, perceptions, ideas, volition, and emotion, in short the whole inner and outer world, are composed of a small number of homogeneous elements connected in relations of varying evanescence or permanence. Usually, these elements are called sensations. But as vestiges of a one-sided theory inhere in that term, we prefer to speak simply of *elements*, as we have already done. The aim of all research is to ascertain the mode of connexion of these elements.[1]

II.

That in this complex of elements, which fundamentally is *one*, the boundaries of bodies and of the ego do not admit of being established in a manner definite and sufficient for all cases, has already been remarked. The comprehending of the elements that

[1] Compare the note at the conclusion of my treatise, *Die Geschichte und die Wurzel des Satzes der Erhaltung der Arbeit*, Prague, Calve, 1872.

are most intimately connected with pleasure and pain, under one ideal mental-economical unity, the ego, is a work of the highest significance for the intellect in the functions which it performs for the pain-avoiding, pleasure-seeking will. The delimitation of the ego, therefore, is instinctively effected, is rendered familiar, and possibly becomes fixed through heredity. Owing to their high practical value, not only for the individual, but for the entire species, the composites "ego" and "body" assert instinctively their claims, and operate with all the power of natural elements. In special cases, however, in which practical ends are not concerned, but where knowledge is an object in itself, the delimitation in question may prove to be insufficient, obstructive, and untenable.[1]

The primary fact is not the *I*, the ego, but the elements (sensations). The elements *constitute* the *I*. *I* have the sensation green, signifies that the element green occurs in a given complex of other elements (sensations, memories). When *I* cease to have the sensation green, when *I* die, then the elements no longer

---

[1]Similarly, *esprit de corps*, class bias, national pride, and even the narrowest minded local patriotism may have a high value, *for certain purposes* But such attitudes will not be shared by the broad-minded inquirer, at least not in moments of research. All such egoistic views are adequate only for practical purposes. Of course, even the inquirer may succumb to habit. Trifling pedantries and nonsensical discussions, the cunning appropriation of others' thoughts, with perfidious silence as to the sources, the metaphorical dysphagia suffered when recognition must be given, and the crooked illumination of others' performances when this is done, abundantly show that the scientist and scholar have also the battle of existence to fight, that the ways of science still lead to the mouth, and that the *pure* quest of knowledge in our present social conditions is still an ideal.

occur in their ordinary, familiar way of association. That is all. Only an ideal mental-economical unity, not a real unity, has ceased to exist.[1]

If a knowledge of the connexion of the elements (sensations) does not suffice us, and we ask, *Who* possesses this connexion of sensations, *Who* experiences the sensations? then we have succumbed to the habit of subsuming every element (every sensation) under some *unanalysed* complex, and we are falling back imperceptibly upon an older, lower, and more limited point of view.[2]

[1] The ego is not a definite, unalterable, sharply-bounded unity. None of these attributes are important; for all vary even within the sphere of individual life; in fact their alteration is even sought after by the individual. *Continuity* alone is important. This view accords admirably with the position which Weismann has recently reached by biological investigations. ("Zur Frage der Unsterblichkeit der Einzelligen," *Biolog. Centralbl.*, Vol. IV., Nos. 21, 22; compare especially pages 654 and 655, where the scission of the individual into two *equal* halves is spoken of.) But this continuity is only a means of predisposing and of conserving what is contained in the ego. This content and not the ego is the principal thing. This content, however, is not confined to the individual. With the exception of some insignificant and valueless personal memories, it remains preserved in *others* even after the death of the individual. The *ego* is unsavable. It is partly the knowledge of this fact, partly the fear of it, that has given rise to the many extravagances of pessimism and optimism, and to numerous religious and philosophical absurdities. In the long run we shall not be able to close our eyes to this simple truth, which is the immediate outcome of psychological analysis. We shall then no longer place so high a value upon the ego, which even during the individual life greatly changes, and which, in sleep or during absorption in some idea, just in our very happiest moments, may be partially or wholly absent. We shall then be willing to renounce *individual* immortality, and not place more value upon the subsidiary elements than upon the principal ones. In this way we shall arrive at a freer and more enlightened view of life, which will preclude the disregard of other egos and the over-estimation of our own. [It will be seen from the above remarks that I consider that form of immortality alone as possessing reality and worth, which, with others, Dr. Paul Carus upholds, and which may be found in his discussions in *The Monist*, *The Open Court, Fundamental Problems*, etc.—Mach, 1895.]

[2] The habit of treating the unanalysed ego-complex as an indiscerptible unity frequently assumes in science remarkable forms. First, the nervous

The so-called unity of consciousness is not an argument in point. Since the apparent antithesis of *real* world and *perceived* world is due entirely to our mode of view, and no actual gulf exists between them, a rich and variously interconnected content of consciousness is in no respect more difficult to understand than a rich and diversified interconnexion of the world.

If we regard the ego as a *real* unity, we become involved in the following dilemma : either we must set over against the ego a world of unknowable entities (which would be quite idle and purposeless), or we must regard the whole world, the egos of other people included, as comprised in our own ego (a proposition to which it is difficult to yield serious assent).

But if we take the ego simply as a *practical* unity, put together for purposes of provisional survey, or

system is separated from the body as the seat of the sensations. In the nervous system again, the brain is selected as the organ best fitted for this end, and finally, to save the supposed psychical unity, a *point* is sought in the brain as the seat of the soul. But such crude conceptions are hardly fit even to foreshadow the roughest outlines of what future research will do for the connexion of the physical and the psychical. The fact that the different organs of sensation and memory are physically *connected* with, and can be readily *excited* by, one another, is probably the foundation of the "psychical unity."

I once heard the question seriously discussed, "How the percept of a large tree could find room in the little head of a man?" Now, although this "problem" is no problem, yet it renders us vividly sensible of the absurdity that can be committed by thinking sensations spatially into the brain. When I speak of the sensations of *another* person, those sensations are, of course, not exhibited in my optical or physical space; they are mentally added, and I conceive them *causally*, not spatially, annexed to the brain observed or represented. When I speak of *my own* sensations, these sensations do not exist spatially in my head, but rather my "head" *shares* with them the same spatial field, as was explained above. (Compare the remarks on Fig. 1.)

[The extent to which the old notion of the soul still pervades modern physiological research, the purpose of which is precisely to overcome that ancient view, may be learned from Hauptmann's *Metaphysik in der Physiologie,* Dresden, 1893, with whose remarks I am in general accord.—Mach. 1895.]

simply as a more strongly coherent group of elements, less strongly connected with other groups of this kind, questions like those above discussed will not arise and research will have an unobstructed future.

In his philosophical notes Lichtenberg says : "We become conscious of certain percepts that are not dependent upon us ; of others that we at least think are dependent upon us. Where is the border-line? We know only the existence of our sensations, percepts, and thoughts. We should say, *It thinks,* just as we say, *It lightens.* It is going too far to say *cogito,* if we translate *cogito* by *I think.* The assumption, or postulation, of the ego is a mere practical necessity." Though the method by which Lichtenberg arrived at this result is somewhat different from ours, we must nevertheless give our full assent to his conclusion.

12.

Bodies do not produce sensations, but complexes of sensations (complexes of elements) make up bodies. If, to the physicist, bodies appear the real, abiding existences, whilst sensations are regarded merely as their evanescent, transitory show, the physicist forgets, in the assumption of such a view, that all bodies are but thought-symbols for complexes of sensations (complexes of elements). Here, too, the *elements* form the real, immediate, and ultimate foundation, which it is the task of physiological research to investigate. By the recognition of this fact, many points of psychology and physics assume more distinct and more economical forms, and many spurious problems are disposed of.

For us, therefore, the world does not consist of mysterious entities, which by their interaction with another, equally mysterious entity, the ego, produce sensations, which alone are accessible. For us, colors, sounds, spaces, times, . . . are the ultimate elements, whose given connexion it is our business to investigate.[1] In this investigation we must not allow our-

[1] I have always felt it as a stroke of special good fortune, that early in life, at about the age of fifteen, I lighted, in the library of my father, on a copy of Kant's *Prolegomena zu jeder künftigen Metaphysik.* The book made at the time a powerful and ineffaceable impression upon me, the like of which I never afterward experienced in any of my philosophical reading. Some two or three years later the superfluous rôle played by "the thing in itself" abruptly dawned upon me. On a bright summer day under the open heaven, the world with my ego suddenly appeared to me as *one* coherent mass of sensations, only more strongly coherent in the ego. Although the actual working out of this thought did not occur until a later period, yet this moment was decisive for my whole view. I had still to struggle long and hard before I was able to retain the new conception in my specialty. With the valuable parts of physical theories we necessarily absorb a good dose of false metaphysics, which it is very difficult to sift out from what deserves to be preserved, especially when those theories have become very familiar to us. At times, too, the traditional, instinctive views would arise with great power and place impediments in my way. Only by alternate studies in physics and in the physiology of the senses, and by historico-physical investigations (since about 1863), and after having endeavored in vain to settle the conflict by a physico-psychological monadology, have I attained to any considerable firmness in my views. I make no pretensions to the title of philosopher. I only seek to adopt in physics a point of view that need not be changed the moment our glance is carried over into the domain of another science ; for, ultimately, all must form one whole. The molecular physics of to-day certainly does not meet this requirement. What I say I have probably not been the *first* to say. I also do not wish to offer this exposition of mine as a special achievement. It is rather my belief that every one will be led to a similar view, who makes a careful survey of any extensive body of knowledge. Avenarius, with whose works I recently became acquainted, approaches my point of view (*Philosophie als Denken der Welt nach dem Princip des kleinsten Kraftmasses,* 1876). Also Hering, in his paper on *Memory* (*Almanach der Wiener Akademie.* 1870, p. 258 ; English translation, O. C. Pub. Co., Chicago, 1895), and J. Popper in his beautiful book, *Das Recht zu leben und die Pflicht zu sterben* (Leipsic, 1878, p. 62), have advanced allied thoughts. Compare also my paper, *Ueber die ökono-*

selves to be impeded by such intellectual abridgments
and delimitations as body, ego, matter, mind, etc.,
which have been formed for special, practical purposes
and with wholly provisional and limited ends in view.
On the contrary, the fittest forms of thought must be
created in and by that research *itself*, just as is done
in every special science.   In place of the traditional,
instinctive ways of thought, a freer, fresher view, con-
forming to developed experience, must be substituted.

13.

Science always takes its origin in the adaptation of
thought to some definite field of experience.   The results of the adaptation are thought-elements, which
are able to represent the field.   The outcome, of
course, is different, according to the character and extent of the province surveyed.   If the province of experience in question is enlarged, or if several provinces
heretofore disconnected are united, the traditional,
familiar thought-elements no longer suffice for the extended province.   In the struggle of acquired habit
with the effort after adaptation, *problems* arise, which
disappear when the adaptation is perfected, to make
room for others which have arisen in the interim.

To the physicist, *quâ* physicist, the idea of "body"

---

mische Natur der physikalischen Forschung (*Almanach der Wiener Akademie*,
1882, p. 179, note; English translation in my *Popular Scientific Lectures*, Chicago, 1895).   Finally let me also refer here to the introduction to W. Preyer's
Reine Empfindungslehre and to Riehl's *Freiburger Antrittsrede*, p. 14. I should
probably have much additional matter to cite as more or less allied to this
line of thought, if my knowledge of the literature were more extensive.

is productive of a real facilitation of view, and is not the cause of disturbance. So, also, the person with purely practical aims, is materially assisted by the idea of the *I* or ego. For, unquestionably, every form of thought that has been designedly or undesignedly constructed for a given purpose, possesses for that purpose a *permanent* value. When, however, research in physics and in psychology meets, the ideas held in the one domain prove to be untenable in the other. From the attempt at mutual adaptation arise the various atomic and monadic theories—which, however, never attain their end. If we regard *sensations*, in the sense above defined, as the *elements of the world*, the problems referred to are practically disposed of, and the *first* and most important adaptation effected. This fundamental view (without any pretension to being a philosophy for all eternity) can at present be adhered to in all provinces of experience; it is consequently the one that accommodates itself with the least expenditure of energy, that is, more economically than any other, to the present *temporary collective state of knowledge*. Furthermore, in the consciousness of its purely economical office, this fundamental view is eminently tolerant. It does not obtrude itself into provinces in which the current conceptions are still adequate. It is ever ready, upon subsequent extensions of the domain of experience, to yield the field to a better conception.

The philosophical point of view of the average

man—if that term may be applied to the naïve realism
of the ordinary individual—has a claim to the highest
consideration.   It has arisen in the process of im-
measurable time without the conscious assistance of
man.   It is a product of nature, and is preserved and
sustained by nature.   Everything that philosophy has
accomplished—the *biological* value of every advance,
nay, of every error, admitted—is, as compared with
it, but an insignificant and ephemeral product of art.
The fact is, every thinker, every philosopher, the moment he is forced to abandon his narrow intellectual
province by practical necessity, immediately returns
to the universal point of view held by all men in common.[1]

To discredit this point of view is not then the purpose of the foregoing "introductory remarks."   The
task which we have set ourselves is simply to show *why*
and to what *purpose* for the greatest portion of life we
hold it, and *why* and for what *purpose* we are provisorily
obliged to abandon it.   No point of view has absolute,
permanent validity.   Each has importance only for
some given end.[2]

[1] [Molière's scourged philosopher (in *Le Mariage forcé*) does not say, It
seems to me that I am pummelled, but, I *am* pummelled.—1895.]

[2] [A kindred view will be found in Avenarius (*Kritik der reinen Erfah-
rung*, and *Der menschliche Weltbegriff*).   Avenarius has also undertaken the
commendable task of explaining the development of philosophy on the basis
of the facts furnished by the history of civilisation.   For a further development of this view, which was evoked by a correspondence with Dr. Paul
Carus, see the Appendix to this volume.—1895.]

THE CHIEF POINTS OF VIEW FOR THE INVESTIGATION OF THE SENSES.

WE WILL now take, from the point of view attained, a broad and general survey of the special problems that will engage our attention.

When once the inquiring intellect has gained, through adaptation, the habit of connecting two things, A and B, in thought, it always thereafter seeks to retain this habit, even where the circumstances are slightly altered. Wherever A makes its appearance, B is added in thought. The principle here formulated, which has its root in an effort for economy, and is particularly noticeable in the work of great investigators, may be termed the *principle of continuity*.

Every observed variation in the connexion of A and B which is sufficiently large to be noticed makes itself felt as a disturbance of the above-mentioned habit, and continues to do so until the latter is sufficiently modified to eliminate the disturbance. We have become accustomed to seeing light deflected in

passing from air to glass, and *vice versa*. But the de-
flexion differs noticeably in different cases, and the
habit gained in some cases cannot be carried over undisturbed to new cases, until we are prepared to asso-
ciate with every particular angle of incidence a particular angle of refraction—a condition satisfied by
the discovery of the so-called law of refraction, or by
acquirement of familiarity with the rule contained in
the same. Thus another and modifying principle confronts that of continuity; we will call it the *principle
of sufficient determinateness,* or *sufficient differentiation.*

The joint action of the two principles may be very
well illustrated by a further analysis of the example
cited.   In order to deal with the phenomena exhibited
in the change of color of light, the idea of the law of
refraction must still be retained, but with every particular color a particular index of refraction must be
associated. We soon perceive that with every particular temperature also, a particular index of refraction must be associated; and so on.

In the end, this process leads to temporary con-
tentment and satisfaction, the two things A and B
being conceived as so connected that to every observable change of the one there corresponds a dependent
change of the other.   It may happen that A as well
as B is conceived as a complex of components, and
that to every particular component of A a particular
component of B corresponds. This occurs, for example, when B is a spectrum, and A the correspond-

ing sample of a compound to be tested, in which case
to every component part of the spectrum one of the
components of the matter volatilised before the spec-
troscope is referred, independently of the others. Only
through complete familiarity with this relation can the
principle of sufficient determinateness be satisfied.

2.

Suppose, now, that we are considering a color-
sensation *B*, not in its dependence on *A*, the heated
matter tested, but in its dependence on the elements
of the retinal process, *N*. In such case, not the *kind*
but only the *direction* of the investigation is changed.
None of the preceding observations lose their force,
and the principles to be followed remain the same.
And this holds good, of course, of all sensations.

Now, sensation may be analysed in itself, immediately, that is, psychologically (which was the course
adopted by Johannes Müller), or the co-ordinate physical (physiological) processes may be investigated according to the methods of physics (the course usually
preferred by the modern school of physiologists), or,
finally, the connexion of psychologically observable
data with the corresponding physical (physiological)
processes may be followed up—a mode of procedure
which will carry us farthest, since in this method observation is directed to all sides, and one investigation
serves to support the other. We shall endeavor to attain
this last-named end wherever it appears practicable.

This being our object, then, it is evident that the principle of continuity and that of sufficient determinateness can be satisfied only on the condition that with the same B (this or that sensation) is always associated the same N (the same nerve-process), and for every observable change of B a corresponding change of N is discoverable.   If B is psychologically analysable into a number of independent components, then we shall rest satisfied only on the discovery, in N, of such components as correspond to the former.   In a word, for all psychically observable details of B we have to seek the corresponding physical details of N.

We may thus establish a guiding principle for our investigations, which may be termed the *principle of the complete parallelism of the psychical and physical.* According to our fundamental conception, which recognises no gulf between the two provinces (the psychical and the physical), this principle is almost a matter of course; but we may also enunciate it, as I did years ago, without the help of this fundamental conception, as a *heuristic* principle of research.[1]

3.

As the principle is stated in rather abstract form, a few concrete examples may now be given.   Wherever

[1]Compare my paper, *Ueber die Wirkung der räumlichen Vertheilung des Lichtreizes auf die Netzhaut (Sitzungsberichte der Wiener Akademie*, Vol. LII., 1865); further *Reichert's und Dubois' Archiv*, 1865, p. 634, and *Grundlinien der Lehre von den Bewegungsempfindungen* (Leipsic : Engelmann, 1875, p. 63). The principle is also implicitly contained in an article of mine in Fichte's *Zeitschrift für Philosophie*, Vol. XLVI., 1865, p. 5.

I have a sensation of space, whether through the sensation of sight or through that of touch, or in any other way, I am obliged to assume the presence of a nerve-process in all cases the same in kind. For all time-sensations, also, I must suppose like nerve-processes.

If I see figures which are the *same in size and shape* but differently colored, I seek, in connexion with the different color-sensations, certain identical space-sensations with their appurtenant identical nerve-processes. If two figures are *similar* (that is, if they yield partly identical space-sensations) then the appurtenant nerve-processes contain partly identical components. If two different melodies have the same rhythm, then, side by side with the different tone-sensations exists in both cases an identical time-sensation with identical appurtenant nerve-processes. If two melodies of different pitch are identical, then the tone-sensations as well as their physical conditions, have, in spite of the different pitch, identical constituents. If the seemingly limitless multiplicity of color-sensations is susceptible of being reduced, by psychological analysis (self-observation), to six elements (fundamental sensations), a like simplification may be expected for the system of nerve-processes. If our system of space-sensations appears in the character of a threefold manifoldness, its system of co-ordinated nerve-processes will likewise present itself as such.

4.

This principle has, moreover, always been more or less consciously, more or less consistently, followed.

For example, when Helmholtz assumes for every tone-sensation a special nerve-fibre in the ear (with its appurtenant nerve-process), when he resolves clangs, or compound sounds, into tone-sensations, when he refers the affinity of compound tones to the presence of like tone-sensations (and nerve-processes),[1] we have in this method of procedure a practical illustration of our principle.   Merely its application is not complete, as will be later shown.   Brewster,[2] guided by a psychological but defective analysis of color-sensations, and by imperfect physical experiments,[3] was led to the view that, corresponding to the three sensations, red, yellow, and blue, there existed likewise physically only three kinds of light, and that, therefore, Newton's assumption of an unlimited number of kinds of light, with a continuous series of refractive indices, was erroneous.

[1] Helmholtz, *Die Lehre von den Tonempfindungen.*   Braunschweig : Vieweg, 1863.   English translation by Alex. J. Ellis.   London : Longmans, Green, & Co.

[2] Brewster, *A Treatise on Optics*, London, 1831.   Brewster regarded the red, yellow, and blue light as extending over the whole solar spectrum, though distributed there with varying intensity, so that, to the eye, red appears at both ends (the red and the violet), yellow in the middle, and blue at the end of greater refrangibility.

[3] Brewster believed that he was able to alter by absorption the nuances of the spectrum—colors regarded by Newton as simple—a result which, if correct, would really destroy the Newtonian conception.   He experimented, however, as Helmholtz (*Physiological Optics*) has shown, with an impure spectrum.

Brewster might easily fall into the error of regarding green as a compound sensation. But had he reflected that color-sensation may make its appearance entirely without physical light, he would have confined his conclusions to the nerve-process and left untouched Newton's assumptions in the province of physics, which are as well founded as his own. Thomas Young corrected this error. He perceived that an unlimited number of kinds of physical light with an uninterrupted series of refractive indices (and wave-lengths) were compatible with a small number of color-sensations and nerve-processes, that a discrete number of color-sensations did answer to the continuum of deflexions in the prism (to the continuum of the space-sensations). But even Young did not apply the principle with full consciousness or strict consistency, wholly apart from the fact that he allowed himself to be misled, in his psychological analysis, by physical prejudices. Young, too, first assumed, as fundamental sensations, red, yellow, and blue, for which he later substituted red, green, and violet—misled, as Alfred Mayer, of Hoboken, has admirably shown,[1] by a physical error of Wollaston's.

[1] *Philosophical Magazine*, February, 1876, p. 111. Wollaston was the first to notice (1802) the dark lines of the spectrum, later named after Fraunhofer, and believed that he saw his narrow spectrum divided by the strongest of these lines into a red, a green, and a violet part. He regarded these lines as the dividing lines of the physical colors. Young took up this conception, and substituted for his fundamental sensations red, yellow, and blue, the colors red, green, and violet. In his first conception, Young regarded green as a composite sensation, in his second, both green and violet as simple. The questionable results which psychological analysis may thus yield, are well calculated to destroy belief in its usefulness in general. But we must not forget that there is no principle in the application of which error is excluded.

The direction in which the theory of color-sensation, which has reached a high degree of perfection through Hering, has still to be modified, was pointed out by me many years ago in another place.[1]

Here, too, practice is determinative. The circumstance that the physical conditions of sensation almost always give rise to composite sensations, and that the components of sensation seldom make their appearance separately, renders psychological analysis very difficult. Thus, green is a simple sensation; a given pigment or spectrum green, however, will as a rule excite also a concomitant yellow or blue sensation, and thus favor the erroneous idea (based upon the results of pigment-mixing) that the sensation of green is compounded of yellow and blue. Careful physical study, therefore, is also an indispensable requisite of psychological analysis. On the other hand, physical observation must not be overestimated. The mere observation that a yellow and blue pigment mixed, yield a green pigment, cannot alone determine the perception of yellow and blue in green, unless one or the other color is actually contained in it. Certainly no one sees yellow and blue in white, although, as a fact, spectrum-yellow and spectrum-blue mixed give white.

[1] I will here condense into a note what I have to say concerning the treatment of the theory of color-sensation. We frequently meet with the assertion, in recent works, that the six fundamental color-sensations, white, black, red, green, yellow, blue, which Hering adopted, were first proposed by Leonardo da Vinci, and later by Mach and Aubert. That the assertion with regard to Leonardo da Vinci was founded upon an error appeared to me, from the very first, in view of the conceptions prevalent at his time, highly probable. Let us hear what he himself says in his *Book of Painting* (Nos. 254 and 255 in the translation of Heinrich Ludwig, *Quellenschriften zur Kunstgeschichte*, Vienna, Braumüller, 1882, Vol. XVIII). "254. Of simple colors there are six. The first of these is white, although philosophers admit neither white nor black into the number of colors, since the one is the cause of colors, the other of their absence. But, *inasmuch as the painter cannot do without them*, we shall include these two also among the other colors and say that white in this classification is the first among the simple colors, yellow the second, green the third, blue the fourth, red the fifth, black the sixth. And the white we will let represent the light, without which one can see no color, the yellow the earth, the green the water, blue the air, red fire, and black the darkness which is found above the element of fire, because in that place there is no matter or solid substance upon which the sunbeams can exert their force, and which as a result they might illumine." "255. Blue and green are not simple colors by themselves. For blue is composed of light and darkness, as, the blue of the air, which is made up of the most perfect black and perfectly pure white." "Green is composed of a simple and a composite color, namely, of yellow and blue." This will suffice to show that Leonardo da Vinci is concerned partly with observations concerning pigments, partly with conceptions of natural philosophy, but not with the subject of fundamental color-sensations. The many remarkable and subtle scientific observations of all sorts which are contained in Leonardo da Vinci's book

The examples adduced will suffice to explain the significance of the above-enunciated principle of inquiry, and at the same time to show that this principle is not entirely new. In formulating the principle, years ago, I had no other object than that of setting clearly before *my own* mind a truth which I had long instinctively felt.

5.

As we recognise no real gulf between the physical and the psychical, it is a matter of course that, in the study of the sense-organs, general physical as well as special biological observations may be employed.

lead to the conviction that the artists, and among them especially he himself, were the true forerunners of the great scientists who came soon afterwards. These men were obliged to understand nature in order to reproduce it agreeably; they observed themselves and others in the interest of pure pleasure. Yet Leonardo was far from being the author of all the discoveries and inventions which Groth, for example, (*Leonardo da Vinci als Ingenieur und Philosoph*, Berlin, 1874,) ascribes to him. My own scattered remarks concerning the theory of color-sensation, were perfectly clear. I assumed the fundamental sensations white, black, red, yellow, green, blue, and six different corresponding (chemical) processes (not nerve-fibres) in the retina. (Compare *Reichert's und Dubois' Archiv*, 1865, p. 633, et seq.) As a physicist, I was of course familiar with the relation of the complementary colors. My conception, however, was that the two complementary processes together excited a new—the white—process. (*Loc. cit.*, p. 634.) I gladly acknowledge the great advantages of Hering's theory. They consist for me in the following. First, the black process is regarded as a *reaction* opposing the white process; I can appreciate all the more the facilitation involved in this conception, as it was just the relation of black and white that for me presented the greatest difficulty. Further, red and green, as also yellow and blue, are regarded as antagonistic processes which do not produce a new process, but mutually annihilate each other. According to this conception white is not subsequently produced but is already present beforehand, and still remains on the annihilation of a color by the complementary color. The only point that still dissatisfies me in Hering's theory is that it is difficult to perceive why the two opposed processes of black and white may be simultaneously produced and simultaneously felt, while such is not the case with red-green and blue-yellow. Compare also my paper, previously cited, in the *Sitzungsberichte der Wiener Akademie*, Vol. 52, 1865, October.

Much that appears to us difficult of comprehension when we draw a parallel between a sense-organ and a physical apparatus, is rendered quite obvious in the light of the theory of evolution, simply by assuming that we are concerned with a living organism with particular memories, particular habits and manners, which owe their origin to a long and eventful race-history. I shall condense what I have to say on this subject into a footnote of some length.[1]   Even teleological

[1] The idea of applying the theory of evolution to physiology in general, and to the physiology of the senses in particular, was advanced, prior to Darwin, by Spencer (1855). It received an immense impetus through Darwin's book *The Expression of the Emotions.* Later, Schuster discussed the question whether there were "inherited ideas" in the Darwinian sense. I, too, expressed myself in favor of the application of the idea of evolution to the theory of the sense-organs (*Sitzungsberichte der Wiener Akademie*, October, 1866). One of the finest and most instructive discussions, in the way of a psychologico-physiological application of the theory of evolution, is to be found in the Academic Anniversary Address of Hering, *On Memory as a General Function of Organised Matter*, 1870, (English translation, Open Court Publishing Company, Chicago, 1895). As a fact, memory and heredity *are* nearly embraced under one concept if we reflect that *organisms*, which were part of the parent-body, *emigrate* and become the basis of new individuals. Heredity is rendered almost as intelligible to us by this thought as, for example, is the fact that Americans speak English, or that their state-institutions much resemble the English, etc. The problem involved in the fact that organisms possess memory, a property which is apparently lacking to inorganic matter, is, of course, not removed by this insight, but still exists.—Recently Weismann (*Ueber die Dauer des Lebens*) has conceived *death* as a phenomenon of heredity. This admirable book, also, contributes greatly to our enlightenment. The difficulty which might be found in the fact that a trait which can make its appearance in the parent-organism only after the process of inheritance is ended should be subject to inheritance, lies probably only in the manner of statement. It disappears when we consider that the power of the cells of the body to multiply can increase, as Weismann shows, only at the cost of the increase of the germ-cells. Accordingly, we may say that greater length of life on the part of the cell-society and lessened propagation are two phenomena which mutually condition each other.—While a student at the Gymnasium, I heard it stated that plants from the Southern Hemisphere bloom in our latitudes, when it is spring in their native place. I recall clearly the mental shock which this communication caused me. If it is true, we have actually a case of plant-memory. The so-called reflex actions of animals may be explained in a natural manner as phenomena of memory outside the organ

conceptions, as aids to investigation, are not to be shunned. It is true, our comprehension of the facts of reality is not enhanced by referring them to an un-

of consciousness. I was a witness of a very remarkable phenomenon of this kind—in 1865, I think—with Rollett, who was experimenting with pigeons whose brains had been removed. These animals drank whenever their feet were placed in a cold liquid, whether the latter was water, mercury, or sulphuric acid. Now since a bird must ordinarily wet its feet when it seeks to quench its thirst, the conception arises quite naturally that we have to do here with a habit adapted to an end, which is conditioned by the mode of life and fixed by inheritance, and which, even when consciousness is eliminated, takes place with the precision of clock-work on the application of the stimulus appropriate to its excitation. Goltz, in his remarkable book *Die Nervencentren des Frosches*, and in later writings, has described many phenomena of the sort.—I will relate, also, in this connexion, some other experiences which I recall with a great deal of pleasure. In the autumn vacation of 1873, my little boy brought me a sparrow a few days old, which had fallen from its nest, and desired to raise it. But the matter was not so easy. The little animal could not be induced to swallow, and would certainly soon have fallen a victim to the indignities that would have been unavoidable in feeding it by force. I then fell into the following train of thought: "Whether or not the Darwinian theory is correct, the new-born child would certainly perish if it had not the perfected organs and inherited impulse to suck, which are brought into activity quite automatically and mechanically by the appropriate excitation. Something similar (in another form) must exist likewise in the case of the bird." I exerted myself to discover the appropriate excitation. A small insect was stuck upon a sharp stick and swung rapidly about the head of the bird. Immediately the bird opened its bill, beat its wings, and eagerly devoured the proffered food. I had discovered the right excitation for setting the impulse and the automatic movement into activity. The animal grew perceptibly stronger and greedier, it began to snatch at the food, and once seized an insect that had accidentally fallen from the stick to the table; from that time on it ate, without ceremony, of itself. In proportion as its intellect developed, the required amount of excitation decreased. On reaching independence, the animal took on, little by little, all the characteristic ways of sparrows, which it certainly had not learnt by itself. By day (during full intellectual activity) it was very trustful and friendly. In the evening, other phenomena were exhibited. The creature grew timid. It always sought out the highest places in the room, and would become quiet only when it was prevented by the ceiling from going higher. Here again we have an inherited habit adapted to an end. On the coming of darkness, the demeanour of the animal changed totally. When approached, it ruffled its feathers, began to hiss, and showed every appearance of terror and real physical fear of ghosts. Nor is this fear without its reasons and its purpose in a creature which, under normal circumstances, may at any moment be devoured by some monster.

This last observation strengthened me in an opinion already formed, that the superstition of my children did not have its source in nursery tales, which were carefully excluded from them, but was innate. One of my children

known World-Purpose, itself problematic. Nevertheless, the question as to the value that a given function
has for the existence of an organism, or as to what are

would regard with anxiety an arm-chair, which stood in the shadow; another
carefully avoided, in the evening, a coal-hod by the stove, especially when
this stood with raised cover, resembling open jaws. The fear of spirits is the
true mother of religions. Neither scientific analysis nor the careful historical criticism of a David Strauss, as applied to myths, which, for the strong
intellect, are refuted even before they are invented, will all at once do away
with and banish these things. Habits which have so long answered, and in a
measure still answer, to actual economic needs (fear of a worse, hope of a
better), will long continue to exist in mysterious and uncontrollable instincts
of the brain. Just as the birds on uninhabited islands (according to Darwin)
learn the fear of man only after the lapse of generations, so we shall unlearn,
only after many generations, that useless habit known as the creeping of flesh.
Every presentation of Faust may teach us the extent to which we are still in
secret sympathy with the conceptions of the age of witchcraft.—I will here
relate one other curious fact, for the knowledge of which I am indebted to my
father (an enthusiastic Darwinian and in the latter part of his life land-pro-
prietor in Carniola). My father occupied himself much with silk-culture,
raised the yami-mai in the open oak woods, etc. The ordinary mulberry silk-
worm has, for many generations, been raised indoors, and has become ex-
ceedingly helpless and dependent. When the time for passing into the chry-
salic state arrives, it is the custom to give the creatures bundles of straw,
upon which they spin their cocoons. Now it one day occurred to my father
not to prepare the usual bundles of straw for a colony of silk-worms. The
result was that the majority of the worms perished, and only a small portion,
the geniuses (those with the greatest power of adaptation) spun their cocoons.
Whether, as my sister believes she has observed, the experiences of one generation are utilised, in noticeable degree, in the very next generation, is a question which must probably be left to further investigation.—From all these remarkable phenomena we need derive no mysticism of the Unconscious. A
memory reaching beyond the individual renders them intelligible.—A psychology in the Spencer-Darwinian sense, founded upon the theory of evolution, but supported by positive investigation of particulars, would yield richer
results than all previous speculation has done.—These observations and conceptions had long been made and written down when Schneider's valuable
work, *Der thierische Wille*, Leipsic, 1880, which contains many that are similar, made its appearance. I agree with the details of Schneider's discussions
almost throughout, although his fundamental conceptions in the realms of natural science with regard to the relation of sensation and physical process, the
significance of the survival of species, etc., are essentially different from
mine, and although I hold, for instance, the distinction between sensation-
impulses and perception-impulses to be quite superfluous.—An important
alteration of our views on heredity may perhaps be expected from Weismann's work, *Ueber die Vererbung*, Jena, 1883 (English translation, *Essays on
Heredity and Kindred Biological Problems*, Oxford: The Clarendon Press,
1889). Weismann regards the inheritance of traits acquired by *use* as highly

its actual contributions to the existence of the same, may be of great assistance in the comprehension of this function.[1] Of course we must not suppose, on this account, as many Darwinians have done, that we

improbable, and finds in the germ-elements and in the selection of the germ-elements the most important factors. We can scarcely withhold our assent to Weismann's arguments, and certainly not refuse recognition to the almost mathematical precision and depth of his presentation of the problem. But that the germ-elements themselves may be altered by outer influences appears to be clearly shown by the formation of new races, which maintain themselves as such, transmit their racial traits, and are themselves, again, capable of alteration, under other circumstances. Accordingly, some influence must certainly be exerted on the germ-plasm by the body which envelops it (as Weismann himself admits). Thus an influence of the individual life upon descendants can certainly not be entirely excluded, even although a direct transmission to the descendants of the results of use in the individual is (according to Weismann) not to be expected.

[I have to add here that I lay great stress on the works of C. Lloyd Morgan, with which I have since become acquainted, and that I agree in almost every point with his expositions.—1895.]

1Such teleological conceptions have often been useful and instructive to me. The remark, for example, that a visible object under varying intensity. of illumination can be recognised as the same only when the sensation excited is in dependence on the *ratio* of the illumination-intensities of object and surroundings, makes intelligible a whole train of organic properties of the eye. We understand through it, also, how the organism, in the interest of its survival, was obliged to adjust itself to the requirement mentioned and to adapt itself to feel the ratios of light-intensity. The so-called law of Weber, or the fundamental psycho-physical formula of Fechner, thus appears not as something fundamental, but as the *explicable* result of organic adjustments. The belief in the universal validity of this law is, naturally, herewith relinquished. I have given the arguments on this point in various papers. (*Sitzungsberichte der Wiener Akademie,* Vol. LII., 1865; *Vierteljahrsschrift für Psychiatrie,* Neuwied and Leipsic, 1868; *Sitzungsberichte der Wiener Akademie,* Vol. LVII., 1868). In the last-named paper, proceeding from the postulate of the parallelism between the psychical and the physical, or, as I then expressed myself, from the *proportionality* between excitation and sensation, I abandoned the *metrical formula* of Fechner (the logarithmic law), and brought forward another conception of the fundamental formula, the validity of which for light-sensation I never disputed. This is apparent beyond all doubt from the mathematical development there found. Thus one cannot say, as Hering has done, that I everywhere take the psycho-physical law as my foundation, if by this is understood the *metrical formula.* How could I maintain the *proportionality* between excitation and sensation at the same time with the *logarithmic* dependence? It was sufficient for me to render *my* meaning clear;—to criticise and contest Fechner's ·law in detail, I had, for many obvious reasons, no need.

have "mechanically explained" a function, when we discover that it is necessary for the survival of the species. Darwin himself is doubtless quite free from this short-sighted conception. The physical means by which a function is developed still remains a physical problem ; while the mode and reason of an organism's voluntary adaptation continues to be a psychological problem. The preservation of the species is only one, though an actual and very valuable, point of departure for inquiry, but it is by no means the last and the highest. Species have certainly been destroyed, and new ones have as certainly arisen. The pleasure-seeking and pain-avoiding will, therefore, is directed perforce beyond the preservation of the species. It preserves the species when it is advantageous to do so ; transforms it when it is advantageous ; and destroys it when its continuance would not be advantageous. Were it directed merely to the preservation of the species, it would move aimlessly about in a vicious circle, deceiving both itself and all individuals. This would be the biological counterpart of the notorious "perpetual motion" of physics.[1]

---

[1] [The same absurdity is committed by the statesman who regards the individual as existing solely for the sake of the State.—1895.]

THE SPACE-SENSATIONS OF THE EYE.

_____

I.

THE tree with its hard, rough, grey trunk, its numberless branches swayed by the wind, its smooth
soft, shining leaves, appears to us at first a single, indivisible whole. In like manner, we regard the sweet,
round, yellow fruit, the warm, bright fire, with its
manifold moving tongues, as a single thing. One name
designates the whole, one word draws forth from the
depths of oblivion all associated memories, as if they
were strung upon a single thread.

The reflexion of the tree, the fruit, or the fire in a
mirror is visible, but not tangible. When we turn our
glance away or close our eyes, we can touch the tree,
taste the fruit, feel the fire, but we cannot see them.
Thus the apparently indivisible thing is separated into
parts, which are not only connected with one another
but are also joined to _other_ conditions. The visible
is separable from the tangible, from that which may
be tasted, etc.

The visible also appears at first sight to be a single

thing.   But we may see a round, yellow fruit together
with a yellow, star-shaped blossom.   A second fruit is
just as round as the first, but is green or red.   Two
things may be alike in color but unlike in form ; they
may be different in color but like in form.   Thus sensations of sight are separable into *color-sensations* and
space-sensations.

2.

Color-sensation, into the details of which we shall
not enter here, is essentially a sensation of favorable
or unfavorable *chemical* conditions of life.   In the process of adaptation to these conditions, color-sensation
may have been developed and modified.[1]   Light in-

[1]Compare Grant Allen, *The Color-Sense* (London: Trübner & Co., 1879).
The attempt of H. Magnus to show a considerable development of the color-
sense within historical times, cannot, I think, be regarded as a felicitous one.
Immediately after the appearance of the writings of Magnus, I corresponded
with a philologist, Prof. F. Polle of Dresden, and both of us
soon came to the conclusion that the views of Magnus could not hold their
own before the critical examination either of natural science or of philology
As each of us left the publication of the results of our discussion to the other
these were never made public. Meantime, however, the matter was disposed of
by E. Krause, and notably by A. Marty. I shall take the liberty of adding only
a few brief remarks. From defects of terminology we cannot infer the absence
of corresponding qualities of sensation. Terms, even to-day, are always indis
tinct, hazy, defective, and few in number, where there is no necessity for
sharp discrimination. The color-terminology of the countryman of to-day-
and his terminology of sensations in general, is no more developed than that
of the Greek poets. The peasants of Marchfeld say, for example, as I have
often proved by personal experience, that salt is "sour," because the expression "salty" is not familiar to them. The terminology of colors must not be
looked for in the poets, but in technical works. And, furthermore, as my col-
league Benndorf has remarked, we must not take an enumeration of vase-
pigments for an enumeration of all colors, as does Mr. Magnus. When we
consider the polychromy of the ancient Egyptians and Pompeiians, when we
take into account the fact that these decorations can scarcely have been produced by the color-blind, when we note that Pompeii was buried in ashes only
seventy years after Virgil's death, whilst Virgil on this theory is supposed to
have been nearly color-blind, the untenability of the whole conception is

troduces organic life. The green chlorophyll and the (complementary) red hæmoglobin play a prominent part in the chemical processes of the plant-body and in the contrary processes of the animal body. The two substances present themselves to us in the most varied modifications of tint. The discovery of the visual purple, observations in photography and photochemistry render the conception of processes of sight as chemical processes permissible. The rôle which color plays in analytical chemistry, in spectrum-analysis, in crystallography, is well known. It suggests a new conception for the so-called vibrations of light, according to which they are regarded, not as mechanical, but as chemical vibrations, as successive union and separation, as an oscillatory process of the same sort that takes place, though only in one direction, in photo-chemical phenomena. This conception, which is substantially supported by recent investigations in abnormal dispersion, accords with the electro-magnetic theory of light. In the case of electrolysis, in fact, chemistry yields the most intelligible conception of the electric

strikingly apparent. Applications of the Darwinian theory are also to be made with caution in another direction. We like to picture to ourselves a condition in which the color-sense is lacking, or in which little color-sense exists, as *preceding* another in which the color-sense is highly developed. For the *beginner* it is natural to proceed from the simple to the complex. But this is not necessarily the path of Nature. The color-sense exists, and it is probably variable. But whether it is being enriched or impoverished—who can tell? Is it not possible that, with the awakening of intelligence and the use of artificial contrivance, the whole development will be devolved on the intellect,—which certainly is chiefly called in play from this point on,—and that the development of the lower organs of man will be relegated to second place?

current, regarding the two components of the electro-
lyte as passing through each other in opposite directions.   It is likely, therefore, that in a future theory
of colors, many biologico-psychological and chemico-
physical threads will be united.

3.

Adaptation to the chemical conditions of life which
manifest themselves in color, renders *locomotion* necessary to a far greater extent than adaptation to those
which manifest themselves through taste and smell.
At least this is so in the case of man, concerning whom
alone we are able to judge with immediacy and certainty.   The close association of space-sensation (a
mechanical factor) with color-sensation (a chemical
factor) is herewith rendered intelligible.   We shall now
proceed to the analysis of space-sensations.

4.

In examining two figures which are alike but differently colored (for example, two letters of the same
size and shape, but of different colors),
we recognise their sameness of form at
the first glance, in spite of the difference of color-sensation.   The sight-per-
ceptions, therefore, must contain some

Fig. 2.

like sensation-components.   These are the space-sensations—which are the same in the two cases.

5.

We will now investigate the character of the space-sensations that physiologically condition the recognition of a figure. First, it is clear that this recognition is not the result of geometrical considerations—which are a matter, not of sensation, but of intellect. On the contrary, the space-sensations in question serve as the starting-point and foundation of all geometry. Two figures may be geometrically. congruent, but physiologically quite different, as is shown by the two ad-

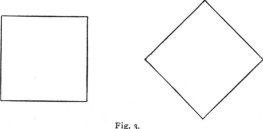

Fig. 3.

joined squares (Fig. 3), which could never be recognised as the same without mechanical and intellectual operations.[1]   A few simple experiments will render us familiar with the relations here involved.   Look at the spot in Fig. 4.   Place the same spot twice or several times in exactly the same position in a row (Fig. 5) ; the result is a peculiar, agreeable impression, and we recognise

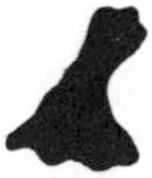

Fig. 4.

[1] Compare my brief paper, *Ueber das Sehen von Lagen und Winkeln*, in the *Sitzungsberichte der Wiener Akademie*, Vol. XLIII., 1861, p. 215.

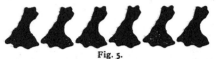

Fig. 5.

at once and without difficulty the identity of all the figures. Turning, however, one spot half way around

Fig. 6.

with respect to the other (Fig. 6), their identity of form is not recognisable without intellectual assistance. On the other hand, if we place two of the

Fig. 7.

spots in positions symmetrical to the median plane of the observer (Fig. 7), the relationship of form is strikingly apparent. But if the plane of symmetry diverges considerably from the median plane of the observer, as in Fig. 8, the affinity of form is rec-

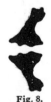

Fig. 8.

ognisable only by turning the figure around or by an *intellectual* act. On the other hand, the affinity of form is again apparent on contrasting with such a spot the same spot rotated through an angle of 180° in the same plane (Fig. 9). In this case we have the so-called centric symmetry.

Fig. 9.

If we reduce all the dimensions of the spot proportionately, we obtain a geometrically similar spot. But as the geometrically congruent is not necessarily physiologically (optically) congruent, nor the geometrically symmetrical necessarily optically symmetrical, analogously the geometrically similar is not necessarily optically similar. If the geometrically similar spots be placed beside each other in the *same* relative positions (Fig. 10), the two will also appear optically similar. Turning one of the spots around destroys the resemblance (Fig. 11). If we substitute for one of the spots a spot symmetrical to the other in respect to the me-- dian plane of the observer (Fig. 12), a symmetrical similarity will be produced which has also an optical

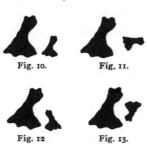

Fig. 10.   Fig. 11.

Fig. 12   Fig. 13.

value. The turning of one of the figures through 180° in its own plane, producing thereby centrically symmetrical similarity, has also a physiologico-optical value (Fig. 13).

6.

In what, now, does the essential nature of optical similarity, as contrasted with geometrical similarity, consist? In geometrically similar figures, all homologous distances are proportional. But this is an affair of the intellect, not of sensation. If we place beside a triangle with the sides *a*, *b*, *c*, a triangle with the sides 2*a*, 2*b*, 2*c*, we do not recognise the simple relation of the two immediately, but intellectually, by measurement. If the similarity is to become optically perceptible, the proper position must be added. That a simple intellectual relationship of two objects does not necessarily condition a similarity of sensation, may be perceived by comparing two triangles having respectively the sides *a, b, c*, and $a+m$, $b+m$, $c+m$. The two triangles do not look at all alike. Similarly all conic sections do not look alike, although all stand in a simple *geometric* relation to each other ; still less do curves of the third order exhibit optical similarity; etc.

7.

The geometrical similarity of two figures is determined by all their homologous lines being proportional or by all their homologous angles being equal. But

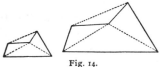

Fig. 14.

to appear optically similar the figures must also be *similarly situated*, that is all their homologous lines must be parallel or, as we prefer to say, have the *same* direction (Fig. 14). The importance of direction for sensation will be evident upon a careful consideration of Fig. 3. By like ness of direction, accordingly, are determined like space-sensations, and these are characteristic of the physiologico-optical similarity of figures.[1]

1 Some twenty years ago, in a society of physicists and physiologists, I proposed for discussion the question, why geometrically similar figures were also optically similar. I remember quite well the attitude taken with regard to this question, which was accounted not only superfluous, but even ludicrous. Nevertheless, I am now as strongly convinced as I was then that the question involves the whole problem of form-vision. That a problem cannot be solved which is not recognised as such is clear. In this non-recognition, however, is manifested, in my opinion, that one-sided mathematico-physical direction of thought, which alone accounts for the opposition, instead of cheerful acceptance, with which the writings of Hering have been received.

We may obtain an idea of the physiological significance of the *direction* of a given straight line or
curve-element, by the following reflexion. Let $y = f(x)$
be the equation of a plane curve. We can read at a
glance the course of the values of dy/dx on the curve,
for they are determined by its slope ; and the eye gives
us, likewise, qualitative information concerning the
values of d^2y/dx^2, for they are characterised by the
curvature. The question naturally presents itself why
can we not arrive at as immediate conclusions concerning the values d^3y/dx^3, d^4y/dx^4, etc. The answer is easy. What we *see* are not the differential
coefficients, which are an intellectual affair, but only
the *direction* of the curve-elements, and the *declination*
of the direction of one curve-element from that of another.

In fine, since we are immediately cognisant of the
similarity of figures lying in similar positions, and are
also able to distinguish without ado the special case of
congruity, therefore our space-sensations yield us information concerning *likeness or unlikeness of directions
and equality or inequality of spatial dimensions.*

8.

It is extremely probable that sensations of space
are produced by the motor apparatus of the eye. Without entering into particulars, we may observe, first,
that the whole apparatus of the eye, and especially
the motor apparatus, is symmetrical with respect to

the median plane of the head.   Hence, symmetrical movements of looking will determine like or approximately like space-sensations. Children constantly confound the letters *b* and *d*, as also *p* and *q*. Adults, too, do not readily notice a change from left to right unless some special points of apprehension for sense or intellect render it perceptible. The symmetry of the motor apparatus of the eye is very perfect. The like excitation of its symmetrical organs would, by itself, scarcely account for the distinction of right and left. But the whole human body, especially the brain, is affected with a slight asymmetry,—which leads, for example, to the preference of one (generally the right) hand, in motor functions. And this leads, again, to a further and better development of the motor functions of the right side, and to a modification of the attendant sensations. After the space-sensations of the eye have become associated, through writing, with the motor functions of the right hand, a confusion of those vertically symmetrical figures with which the art and habit of writing are concerned no longer ensues. This association may, indeed, become so strong that remembrance follows only the accustomed tracks, and we read, for example, the reflexion of written or printed words in a mirror only with the greatest difficulty. The confusion of right and left still occurs, however, with regard to figures which have no motor, but only a purely optical (for example, ornamental) interest. A noticeable difference between right and left must be

felt, moreover, by animals, as in many predicaments
they have no other means of finding their way. The
similarity of sensations connected with symmetrical
motor functions is easily remarked by the attentive
observer. If, for example, supposing my right hand
to be employed, I grasp a micrometer-screw or a key
with my left hand, I am certain (unless I reflect beforehand) to turn it in the wrong direction,—that is, I
always perform the movement which is symmetrical
to the usual movement, confusing the two because of
the similarity of the sensation. The observations of
Heidenhain regarding the reflected writing of persons
hypnotised on one side should also be cited in this
connexion.

With looking upwards and looking downwards,
fundamentally different space-sensations are associated, as ordinary observation will show. This is,
moreover, comprehensible, since the motor apparatus
of the eye is asymmetrical with respect to a horizontal
plane. The direction of gravity is so very decisive
and important for the motor apparatus of the rest of
the body that the same factor has assuredly also found
its expression in the apparatus of the eye, which serves
the rest. It is well known that the symmetry of a
landscape and of its reflexion in water is not felt.
The portrait of a familiar personage, when turned upside down, is strange and puzzling to a person who
does not recognise it intellectually. If we place ourselves behind the head of a person lying upon a couch

and unreflectingly give ourselves up to the impression
which the face makes upon us, we shall find that it is
altogether strange, especially when the person speaks.
The letters b and p, and d and q, are not confused by
children.

Our previous remarks concerning symmetry, similarity, and the rest, naturally apply not only to plane
figures, but also to those in space.   Hence, we have
yet a remark to add concerning the sensation of space-
depth.   Looking at objects afar off and looking at
objects near at hand determine different sensations.
These sensations *must* not be confused, because of the
supreme importance of the difference between near
and far, both for animals and human beings.   They
cannot be confused because the motor apparatus is
asymmetrical with respect to a plane perpendicular to
the direction from front to rear.   The observation that
the bust of a familiar personage cannot be replaced by
the mould in which the bust is cast is quite analogous
to the observations consequent upon the inversion of
objects.

9.

If equal distances and like directions excite like
space-sensations, and directions symmetrical with respect to the median plane of the head excite similar
space-sensations, the explanation of the above-cited
facts is not far to seek.   The straight line has, in all
its elements, the same direction, and everywhere ex-

cites the same space-sensations. Herein consists its æsthetic value. Moreover, straight lines which lie in the median plane or are perpendicular to it are brought into special relief by the circumstance that, through this position of symmetry, they occupy a like position to the two halves of the visual apparatus. Every other position of the straight line is felt as awryness, or as a deviation from the position of symmetry.

The repetition of the same space-figure in the same position conditions a repetition of the same space-sensation. All lines connecting prominent (noticeable) homologous points have the same direction and excite the same sensation. Likewise when merely geometrically similar figures are placed side by side in the same positions, this relation holds. The sameness of the dimensions alone is absent. But when the positions are disturbed, this relation, and with it, the impression of unity—the æsthetic impression—are also disturbed.

In a figure symmetrical with respect to the median plane, *similar* space-sensations corresponding to the symmetrical directions take the place of the *identical* space-sensations. The right half of the figure stands in the same relation to the right half of the visual apparatus as the left half of the figure does to the left half of the visual apparatus. If we alter the sameness of the dimensions, the sensation of symmetrical similarity is still felt. An oblique position of the plane of symmetry disturbs the whole effect.

If we turn a figure through 180°, contrasting it

with itself in its original position, centric symmetry is
produced.   That is, if two pairs of homologous points
be connected, the connecting lines will cut each other
at a point *O*, through which, as their point of bisec-
tion, all lines connecting homologous points will pass.
Moreover, in the case of centric symmetry, all lines of
connexion between homologous points have the same
direction,—a fact which produces an agreeable sensation.   If the sameness of the dimensions is eliminated,
there still remains, for sensation, centrically symmetrical similarity.

Regularity appears to have no special physiological
value, in distinction from symmetry.   The value of
regularity probably lies rather in its *manifold* symmetry,
which is perceptible in more than one *single* position.

10.

The correctness of these observations will be apparent on glancing over the work of Owen Jones—*A
Grammar of Ornament* (London, 1865).   In almost
every plate one finds new and different kinds of symmetry as fresh testimony in favor of the conceptions
above advanced.   The art of decoration, which, like
pure instrumental music, aims at no ulterior end, but
ministers only to pleasure in form (and color), is the
best source of material for our present studies.   Writing is governed by other considerations than that of
beauty.   Nevertheless, we find among the twenty-four
large Latin letters ten which are vertically symmetri-

cal (A, H, I, M, O, T, V, W, X, Y), five which are
horizontally symmetrical (B, C, D, E, K), three which
are centrically symmetrical (N, S, Z), and only six
which are unsymmetrical (F, G, L, P, Q, R).

II.

It is to be remarked again that the geometrical
and the physiological properties of a figure in space
are to be sharply distinguished. The physiological
properties are determined by the geometrical properties coincidently with these, but are not determined
by these solely. On the other hand, physiological
properties very probably gave the first impulse to
geometrical investigations. The straight line doubtless attracted attention not because of its being the
shortest line between two points, but because of
its physiological simplicity. The plane likewise possesses, in addition to its geometrical properties, a special physiologico-optical (æsthetic) value, which claims
notice for it, as will be shown later on. The division
of the plane and of space by right angles has not only
the advantage of producing equal parts, but also an
additional and special symmetry-value. The circumstance that congruent and similar geometrical figures
can be brought into positions where their relationship
is physiologically felt, led, no doubt, to an earlier
investigation of these kinds of geometrical relationship than of those that are less noticeable, such as affinity, collineation, and others. Without the co-ope-

ration of sense-perception and understanding, a scientific geometry is inconceivable. But H. Hankel has admirably shown in his *History of Mathematics* (Leipsic, 1874) that in the Greek geometry the factor of pure understanding, in the Indian, on the other hand, that of sense, very considerably predominated. The Hindus make use of the principles of symmetry and similarity (see, for example, p. 206 of Hankel's book) with a generality which is totally foreign to the Greeks. Hankel's proposition to unite the rigor of the Greek method with the perspicuity of the Indian in a new mode of presentation is well worthy consideration. Furthermore, in so doing, we should only be following in the footsteps of Newton and John Bernoulli, who have made a still more general application of the principle of similitude in mechanics. The advantages that the principle of symmetry affords in the last-named province, I have shown elsewhere.[1]

---

[1] I have given less complete discussions of the leading thoughts of this chapter in the paper already mentioned, *Ueber das Sehen von Lagen und Winkeln* (1861), further in Fichte's *Zeitschrift für Philosophie*, Vol. XLVI., 1865, p. 5 and in *The Forms of Liquids*, and *Symmetry* (1872) now also published in my *Popular Scientific Lectures*, translated by Thomas J. McCormack, Open Court Publishing Co., Chicago, 1894. With regard to the use of the principle of symmetry in mechanics, compare my work *The Science of Mechanics* (1883), translated by Thomas J. McCormack, 1893, Open Court Pub. Co., Chicago. [I must also refer in this place to a work which has since appeared, by J. L. Soret, *Des conditions physiques de la perception du beau*, Geneva, 1892. In this charmingly written book Soret makes extensive applications of the principle of *repetition* of sensations to æsthetics. Applications of this kind I had treated only briefly, as it was not my purpose to write a book on æsthetics. On the other hand, I believe I have penetrated deeper into the physiological and psychological aspect of the principle.—MACH, 1895.]

INVESTIGATION OF SPACE-SENSA-TION CONTINUED.[1]

1.

That space-sensation is connected with motor pro-cesses has long since ceased to be disputed. Opinions differ only as to how this connexion is to be repre-sented.

2.

If two congruent images of different colors fall in succession on the same parts of the retina, they are at once recognised as identical figures. We may, therefore, regard different space-sensations as con-nected with different parts of the retina. But that these space-sensations are not *unalterably* restricted to particular parts of the retina, we perceive on moving

---

[1] To my knowledge, the matter treated in the preceding chapter has not yet been discussed, except in three small works of my own. The considerations of the present chapter, moreover, are, for me, founded upon those of the pre-ceding chapter. I indicate here the methods by which I have myself gotten clear regarding the sensation of space, without laying the least claim to that which has been accomplished by others in this direction, particularly by the theory of Hering. The extensive literature of this subject is, moreover, too imperfectly known to me to give exact references on all points. The point of Hering's theory which I regard as the most important I will especially notice.

our eyes freely and voluntarily, whereby the objects observed do not change their position or form, although their images are displaced on the retina.

If I look straight before me, fixing my eyes upon an object *O*, an object *A*, which is reflected on the retina in *a*, at a certain distance below the point of most distinct vision, appears to me to be situated at a certain height. If I now raise my eyes, fixing them upon *B*, *A* retains its former height. It would neces-

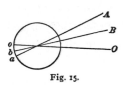

sarily appear lower down if the position of the image on the retina, or the arc *oa*, alone determined the space-sensation. I can raise my glance as far as *A*

Fig. 15.

and farther without a change in this relation. Thus, the physiological process which conditions the *voluntary* raising of the eye, can entirely or partly take the place of the height-sensation, is homogeneous with it, or, in brief, algebraically summationable with it. If I turn my eyeball upward by a slight pressure of the finger, the object *A* actually appears to sink, proportionately to the shortening of the arc *oa*. The same thing happens when, by any other unconscious or involuntary process—for example, through a cramp of the muscles of the eye—the eyeball is turned upward. According to an experience now familiar to opticians for some decades patients with paralysis of the rectus externus reach too far to the right in attempting to grasp objects at the right. Since they need to exert a stronger impulse of the will than persons of sound eyes, in order to fix their glance upon an object to the right, the thought naturally suggests itself that the will to look to the right determines the optical space-sensation "right." Some years ago,[1] I put this observation into the form of an experiment, which every one can try for himself. Let the eyes be turned as far as possible towards the left and two large lumps of moderately hard putty firmly pressed against the right side of each eye-ball. If, now, we attempt to glance quickly to the right, we shall succeed only very imperfectly, owing to the incompletely spherical form of the eyes, and the objects will suffer a strong displacement to the right. Thus the *mere will* to look to the right imparts to the images at certain points of the retina a larger "rightward value," as we may term it for brevity. The experiment is, at first, surprising. It will soon be perceived, however, that both facts—viz., that by voluntarily turning the eyes to the right, objects are not displaced, and that by the forced, involuntary turning of the eyes to the right, objects are displaced to the left—together amount to the same thing. My eye, which I wish to, and cannot, turn to the right, may be regarded as voluntarily turned to the right and compulsorily turned back by an outer force.

[1] Shortly after finishing my *Grundlinien der Lehre von den Bewegungs-empfindungen.*

3.

The will to perform movements of the eyes, or the innervation to the act, is itself the space-sensation. This follows naturally from the preceding consideration.[1] If we have a sensation of itching or pricking in a certain spot, by which our attention is sufficiently secured, we immediately grasp at the spot with the correct amount of movement. In the same manner we turn our eyes with the correct amount of exertion towards an object reflected on the retina, as soon as this exerts a sufficient stimulus to draw our attention. By virtue of organic apparatus and long exercise we hit immediately upon the exact degree of innervation necessary to enable us to fix our eyes upon an object reflected on a certain point of the retina. If the eyes are already turned towards the right, and we begin to give our attention to an object further to the right or the left, a new innervation of the same sort is algebraically added to that already present. A disturbance of the process arises only when extraneous, involuntary innervations or outward moving forces are added to the innervations determined by the will.

4.

Years ago, while occupied with the questions now under discussion, I noticed a peculiar phenomenon,

---

[1] I retain the expression which was first immediately suggested to me, with no intention of forestalling future inquiry.

which has not yet, to my knowledge, been described. In a very dark room we fix our eyes upon a light *A*, and then suddenly look at a light lower down, *B*. At this, the light *A* appears to make a rapid sweep *A A'* (quickly ended) upwards. The light *B*, of course, does the same—but to avoid complications, this is not indicated in the diagram. The sweep is, of course, an after-image, which enters consciousness only on completion, or shortly before completion, of the glance-movement, but—and this is the remark- able point—with po- sitional values that correspond, not to the later, but to the ear- lier innervations and position of the eye. Similar phenomena

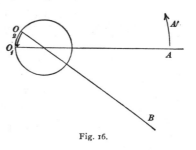

Fig. 16.

are often noticed in experiments with Holtz's elec- trical machine. If the experimenter is surprised by a spark during a glance downwards, the spark often appears high above the electrodes. If it yields a *per- manent* after-image, the latter appears, of course, be- low the electrodes. The preceding phenomena an- swer to the so-called personal equation of astronomers, except that they are confined to the province of sight. By what organic apparatus this relation is determined cannot be decided now, but it is probably of some

value in preventing confusion of position in movements of the eyes.

5.

For the sake of simplicity we have hitherto regarded only the eyes as in motion, and have considered
the head (and the body generally) as at rest.   If, now,
we move the head about without intentionally fixing
the eyes upon any object, the objects seen remain
motionless.   But at the same time another observer
may notice that the eyes, like frictionless, inert masses,
take no part in the turning movements.   Still more

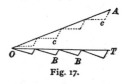

Fig. 17.

noticeable is the phenomenon if
we turn for a considerable time
and with continuous motion about
a vertical axis, in the direction
of the hands of a clock viewed
from above.   In this case, as Breuer has observed, the
open or closed eyes turn, about ten times to a full revo-
lution of the body, in the opposite direction to that of
the clock-hands, with a uniform motion, and as frequently back again in the opposite direction by jerks.
The process is represented in the diagram of Fig. 17.
On OT, the times are laid off as abscissas, the angles
described in the direction of the clock-hands are laid
off as ordinates upwards, and the angles described in
the opposite direction as ordinates downwards.   The
curve OA corresponds to the rotation of the body,
OBB to the relative, and OCC to the absolute, rota-

tion of the eyes. No one, on repeating the experiment, can avoid the conclusion that we are concerned
here with an automatic (unconscious) movement of
the eyes, reflexively excited by the rotation of the
body. How this motion is brought about remains,
naturally, to be investigated. A simple conception
would be that the excitation, uniformly reaching two
antagonistic organs of innervation on the turning of
the body, is answered by one with a uniform stream of
innervation, while the other gives its impulse of innervation only after the lapse of a certain time, like a
filled rain-gauge suddenly overturning. For us it suffices, provisorily, to know that this automatic, unconscious compensational movement of the eye is actually
present.

The slower unconscious compensational movement
of the eye (the jerking motion leaving behind it no optical impression) is thus the cause of the retention of
position by objects seen during the turning of the body
—a thing which is very important for orientation. If,
now, in turning our head, we also voluntarily turn the
eyes in the same direction, fixing them upon one object after another, we must overcompensate the automatic, involuntary innervation by the voluntary innervation. We need the same innervation as if the whole
angle turned through were described by the eye alone.
In this way is explained why, when we turn about, the
whole optical space appears to us a continuity and not
an aggregation of fields of vision ; and why, at the

same time, the optical objects remain stationary. That
which we see of our own body, in turning, we see, for
obvious reasons, optically in motion.

Thus we arrive at the practically valuable conception of our body as in motion in a fixed space. We
understand why it is that, in our numerous turnings
and ramblings in the streets and in buildings, and in
our passive turnings in a wagon or in the cabin of a
ship—yes, even in the dark—we do not lose our sense
of direction, though it is true that the primary co-
ordinates from which we started gradually sink unnoticed into unconsciousness, and we soon begin to
reckon from new objects around us. That peculiar
state of confusion as to locality in which we sometimes find ourselves on suddenly awaking at night,
where we look about helplessly for the window or the
table, is probably due to dreams of movement immediately preceding our awaking.

Similar phenomena to those which manifest themselves on the rotation of the body make their appearance in connexion with the movements of the body
generally. If I move my head or my whole body side-
wise, I do not lose sight of an object on which my
eyes rest. The latter seems to continue motionless,
while the more distant objects undergo a movement in
the same direction as that of the body, the nearer an
opposite, parallactic displacement. The parallactic
displacements to which we are accustomed are perceived, but do not cause us any disturbance and are

correctly interpreted. But in the monocular inversion of a Plateau wire-net, the parallactic displacements, which in the present case are unusual as regards amount and direction, immediately attract the eye, and apparently present to us a revolving object.[1]

6.

When I turn my head, I not only see that part of it turning which I am able to see (as will be immediately understood from the foregoing) but I also *feel* it turning. This is due to the fact that conditions exist in the province of touch which are quite analogous to those in the province of sight.[2] When I reach out my hand to grasp an object, a sensation of touch is combined with a sensation of innervation. If I look towards the object, a luminous sensation is substituted for the sensation of touch. Even where objects are not touched, skin-sensations may always be perceived when the attention is turned to them, and these, combined

[1] Compare my " Beobachtungen über monoculare Stereoscopie " (*Sitzungsberichte der Wiener Akademie*, Vol. LVIII., 1868).

[2] The view that the sense of sight and the sense of touch involve, so to speak, the same space-sense as a common element, was advanced by Locke and contested by Berkeley. Diderot also (*Lettres sur les aveugles*) is of opinion that the space-sense of the blind is altogether different from that of a person who sees. Compare on this point the acute remarks of Dr. Th. Loewy (*Common Sensibles. Die Gemeinideen des Gesichts- und Tastsinnes nach Locke und Berkeley*) with whose results, however, I cannot agree. The circumstance that a man blind from birth does not, after being operated upon, *visually* distinguish the cubes and spheres with which he is familiar from touch proves to my mind nothing at all against Locke and nothing in favor of Berkeley and Diderot. Even persons who see recognise figures that are turned upside down only after much practice. Besides, if Locke were wrong, how could a blind Saunderson have written a geometry intelligible to people gifted with sight. Let a blind man attempt to write a theory of color!

with changing innervations, also yield a conception of our body as in motion, which quite accords with that acquired by optical means.

Thus, in active movements, the skin-sensations are delocalised, as we may briefly express it. In passive movements of the body, reflex, unconscious innervations and movements of compensation make their appearance. In turning round to the right, for example, my skin-sensations are connected with the same innervations as would be combined with the touching of objects in turning to the right. I feel myself turning to the right. If I am passively turned toward the right, the reflex endeavor arises to compensate the turning. I either actually remain standing and feel myself at rest, or I repress the motion toward the left. But for this I need to exert the same voluntary innervation as for an active turning to the right, which has also the same sensation as its result.

7.

At the time when my work on the *Sensations of Movement*[1] was written, I had not yet attained to a thoroughly comprehensive view of the simple relation here described. I encountered, consequently, difficulties in the explanation of certain phenomena, observed by Breuer and myself, which are now easy of explanation, and which I will briefly notice. If an observer

[1] *Grundlinien der Lehre von den Bewegungsempfindungen.* Leipsic: Engelmann, 1875. P. 83.

be shut up in a closed receptacle, and the receptacle be set in rotation toward the right, the same will appear to the observer in rotation, although every ground of inference for relative rotation is wanting. If his eyes perform involuntary, compensatory movements to the left, the images on the retina will be displaced, with the result that he has the sensation of movement toward the right. If, however, he fixes his eyes upon the receptacle, he must voluntarily compensate the involuntary movements, and thus again he is conscious of movement towards the right. It is plain, therefore, that Breuer's explanation of the apparent motion of optical vertigo is correct, and also that this movement cannot be made to disappear by the voluntary fixation of the eyes. The remaining cases of optical vertigo noticed in my work may be disposed of in like manner.[1]

In voluntary forward motion or rotation, we have not only a sensation of every single successive position of the parts of our body, but also the much more simple sensation of movement forward or of turning round. As a fact, we do not form the notion of forward movement from the percepts of the various individual movements of the legs, or at least are not constrained to do so. There are cases, indeed, in which the sensation of forward movement is undoubtedly present while that of the movements of the legs is altogether lack-

---

[1] *Grundlinien der Lehre von den Bewegungsempfindungen.* Leipsic, Engelmann, 1875. P. 83.

ing. This is true, for instance, of a railway-journey,
or even of the thought of such a journey, and may occur also in recalling a distant place, etc. The only
possible explanation of this can be that the *will* to
move *forward* or to *turn about*, which furnishes to the
extremities their motor impulses,— impulses which
may be further modified by particular innervations,—
is of a comparatively *simple* nature. The conditions
existing here are probably similar to, although more
complicated than, those connected with the movements
of the eyes, which Hering has so felicitously interpreted, and to which we shall presently return.

8.

The following experiments and reflexions, which
form a sequel to an earlier publication of mine, will
perhaps assist us in obtaining a correct view of these
phenomena.

If we take our stand upon a bridge, and look fix-
edly at the water flowing beneath, we shall generally
have the sensation of being ourselves at rest, whilst
the water will seem in motion. Prolonged gazing,
however, almost invariably results in the sensation
that suddenly the bridge, with the observer and his
whole environment, begins to move in the direction
opposite to that of the water, while the water assumes
the appearance of being at rest.[1] The *relative* motion

---

[1] As we all know, the most varied forms of the same impression are obtained in the midst of a number of railway trains indiscriminately in motion
and at rest. A short time ago, while making a steamboat excursion on the

of the objects is in both cases the same, and there must therefore be some adequate physiological reason why at one time one, and at another, another part of them is felt to move. In order to investigate the matter at my leisure, I had the simple apparatus constructed which is represented in Fig. 18. An oil-cloth of simple pattern is drawn horizontally over two rollers, two metres long and fixed three metres apart in bearings, and is kept in uniform motion by means of a crank. Across the oil-cloth and about thirty centimetres above it, is stretched a string *ff*, with a knot *K*, which serves as a fixation-point for the eye of the observer stationed at *A*. Now, if the oil-cloth be set

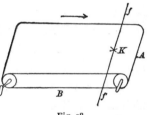

Fig. 18.

in motion in the direction of the arrow, and the observer follow the *pattern* with his eyes, he will see it in motion, himself and his surroundings at rest. On the other hand, if he gazes at the knot, he and the whole room will presently appear in motion in the contrary direction to the arrow, while the oil-cloth will stand still. This change in the aspect of the motion takes more or less time according to the mental condition of the observer, but usually requires only a few seconds. If we once get the knack of it, the two impres-

Elbe, I was astonished at discovering, just before landing, that the ship was standing still and that the whole landscape was moving towards it—an experience that will be readily understood from what follows.

sions may be made to alternate with some rapidity and at will. Every following of the oil-cloth brings the observer to rest, every fixation of K, or non-attention to the oil-cloth, by which its pattern becomes blurred, sets the observer in motion. This phenomenon, of course, must not be confounded with the familiar Plateau-Oppel phenomenon, which is a *local* retinal effect. In the preceding experiment, the entire environment, so far as it is distinctly visible, is in motion, whilst in the latter a moving veil is drawn along in front of the object, which is at rest. The attendant stereoscopic phenomena,—for example, the appearance of the thread and knot underneath the transparent oil-cloth,—are quite immaterial in this connexion.[1]

Before we proceed to the explanation of the experiment, it will be well to introduce a few variations. An observer stationed at B seems, under the same conditions, to be speeding, with all his surroundings, towards the left. We now place above the oil-cloth TT, Fig. 19, a mirror SS, inclined at an angle of 45° to the horizon. We observe the reflexion TT in SS, after having placed on our nose a shade nn, which in-

---

[1] In my book on *Bewegungsempfindungen* (p. 63) I stated that the Plateau-Oppel phenomenon was the result of a *peculiar* process, which was not concerned in the other sensations of movement. I wrote there as follows :

"We must therefore suppose that, during the movement of an image on the retina, a *peculiar* process is excited which is absent during rest, and that in the case of movements in opposite directions, very similar processes are excited in similar organs, processes which are, however, mutually exclusive, so that with the commencement of the one, the other must cease, and with the exhaustion of the one, the other begins."

This statement of mine seems to have been overlooked by S. Exner and Vierordt, who subsequently expressed similar views on the same subject.

tercepts the direct view of *TT* from the eye, *O.* If *TT* moves in the direction of the arrow, while we are looking at *K'*, the reflexion of K, we shall presently fancy ourselves sinking downward with the whole room, whereas if the motion be reversed we shall seem to ascend as if in a balloon.[1] Finally, the experiments with the paper drum, which I have elsewhere described, and to which the following explanation also applies, should be cited here. *None* of these phenomena are *purely optical*, but all are accompanied by unmistakable motor sensations of the whole body.

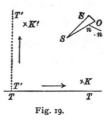

Fig. 19.

9.

What form, now, must our thoughts take on, in order to acquire the simplest explanatory setting for the preceding phenomena? Objects in motion exert, as is well known, a peculiar motor stimulus upon the eye, and draw our attention and look after them. If the eye really follows them, we must assume, from what has gone before, that the objects move. But if the eye is kept at rest, and is forcibly restrained from following the moving objects, the constant stimulus to motion proceeding from the latter must be counterbalanced

[1] Such phenomena often make their appearance quite unsought. As my little daughter was once standing near a window, on a calm winter's day, during a heavy snow-fall, she suddenly cried out that she was rising upward with the whole house.

by an equally constant stream of innervation flowing
to the motor apparatus of the eye, exactly as if the
motionless point on which the eyes rest were moving
uniformly in the opposite direction, and we were following that with our eyes.   But when this process begins, all motionless objects on which the eyes are fast-
ened must appear in motion.   It is obviously unnecessary that this stream of innervation should always be
consciously and deliberately called into action.   All
that is requisite is that it should proceed from the
same centre and by the same paths as intentional fixation.

No special apparatus is necessary for observing
the foregoing phenomena.   They are to be met with
on all hands.   I walk forward by a simple act of the
will.   My legs perform their functions without special
intervention on my part.   My eyes are fixed stead-
fastly upon their goal without suffering themselves to
be drawn aside by the motion of the retinal images
consequent upon progression.   All this is brought
about by a single act of the will, and this act of the
will itself is the sensation of forward movement.   The
same process, or at least a part of it, must also be set
up, if the eyes are made to resist permanently the excitation of a mass of moving objects.   Hence the motor
sensations experienced in the foregoing experiments.

The eyes of a child on a railway-train will be observed to follow almost uninterruptedly and with a
jerking motion the objects outside, which appear to it

to be running. The adult has the same sensation if he will passively yield himself to the natural impressions. If I am riding forwards, the whole space to my left, for obvious reasons, rotates, in the direction of the hands of a watch, about a very distant vertical axis, and the space to my right does the same, but in the opposite direction. Only when I *resist* following the objects with my eyes, does the sensation of forward motion arise.

10.

Without doing violence to the *facts* described in my book on *The Sensations of Movement,* the preceding observations suggest the possibility of modifying the *theoretical view* there taken of the facts, as we shall point out in the following.[1] It is extremely probable

[1] My views regarding the sensations of movement have been repeatedly attacked, as is well known, but invariably the adverse arguments have been aimed solely at the *hypothesis,* to which I attached comparatively little importance. That I am ready and willing to modify my views in accordance with newly discovered facts, the present work will testify. The decision as to how far I am in the right I will cheerfully leave to the future. On the other hand, observations have been made that strongly favor the theory propounded by myself, Breuer, and Brown. To these belong, first, the facts collected by Dr. Guye of Amsterdam (*Du Vertige de Ménière: Rapport lu dans la section d'otologie du congrès périodique international de sciences médicales à Amsterdam,* 1879). Guye observed, in diseases of the middle ear, that reflex turnings of the head were induced when air was blown into the cavity of the tympanum, and found a patient who was able to state exactly the direction and number of the turnings which he had felt during the injection of liquids. —Prof. Crum Brown ("On a Case of Dyspeptic Vertigo," *Proceedings of the Royal Society of Edinburgh,* 1881-1882), has described an interesting case of pathological vertigo observed in himself, which admitted of explanation, as a whole, by the increased intensity and lengthened duration of the sensation incident upon every turning of the body.—But most remarkable of all are the observations of William James ("The Sense of Dizziness in Deaf-Mutes,' *American Journal of Otology,* Vol. IV., 1882). James discovered in deaf-mutes a striking and relatively general insensibility to the dizziness of whirling,

that an organ exists in the head—it may be called the
terminal organ (*TO*)—which reacts upon *accelerations,*

often great uncertainty in their walk when their eyes were closed, and in
many cases an astonishing loss of the sense of direction on being plunged under water, in which case there always resulted alarm and complete uncertainty
as to up and down. These facts speak very strongly in favor of the view, which
naturally follows from my conception, that in deaf-mutes the sense of equilibrium proper is considerably degenerated, and that the two other localising
senses, the sense of sight and the muscular sense, (the latter of which loses
all its points of reference when the weight of the body is neutralised by im-
mersion in water,) are rendered proportionately more necessary.

The view is untenable that we arrive at knowledge of equilibrium and of
movement *solely* by means of the semi-circular canals. On the contrary, it is
extremely probable that lower animals, in whom this organ is entirely wanting, also have sensations of movement. I have not yet been able to under-
take experiments in this direction. But the experiments which Lubbock has
described in his work, *Ants, Bees, and Wasps,* become much more comprehensible to me on the assumption of sensations of movement. As experiments of this sort may be interesting to others, it will not be amiss perhaps to
consider an apparatus which I have briefly described before (*Anzeiger der
Wiener Akademie,* December 30, 1875).

The apparatus serves for the observation of the conduct of animals while
in rapid rotation. Since, however, the view of the animal will necessarily be
effaced by the rotary motion, the passive rotation must be optically nullified
and eliminated, so that the active movements of the animal alone shall be
left and rendered observable. The optical neutralisation of the rotary motion is attained simply by causing a totally reflecting prism to revolve, with
the aid of gearing, above the disk of the whirling machine, about exactly
the same axis, in the same direction, and with half the angular velocity of the
disk.

Fig. 20 gives a view of the apparatus. On the disk of the whirling machine is a glass receiver, *g,* in which the animals to be observed are enclosed.
By means of gearing the eye-piece *o* is made to revolve with half the angular
velocity and in the same direction as *g.* The following figure gives the gearing in a separate diagram. The eye-piece *oo,* and the receiver *gg,* revolve
about the axis *AA,* while a pair of cog-wheels, rigidly connected together, revolve about *BB.* Let the radius of the cog-wheel *aa* be *r;* that of *bb* also *r,*
that of *cc* 2*r*/3, and that of *dd* 4*r*/3, wherewith the desired relation of velocity between *oo* and *gg* is obtained.

In order to centre the apparatus, a mirror *S,* provided with levelling-
screws, is laid upon the bottom of the receiver and so adjusted that, on rotation, the reflexions in it remain at rest. It is then perpendicular to the axis
of rotation. A second small mirror, *S',* in the silvering of which is a small
hole *L,* is so adjusted to the open tube of the eye-piece, with its reflecting surface downward, that, on rotation, the images seen through the hole, in the
mirrored reflexion of *S'* in *S,* remain motionless. Then *S'* stands perpendicular to the axis of the eye-piece. With the aid of a brush we may now mark
upon the mirror *S* a point *P,* whose position is not altered on rotation (a re-

and by means of which we are made aware of movements. But instead of imagining that *special* motor

sult which is easily accomplished after a few trials), and so place the hole in
the mirror S' that it also remains stationary on rotation. In this way points

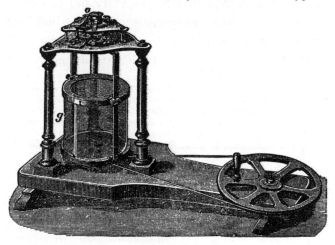

Fig. 20.

on both axes of rotation are found. If now—by means of screws—we so
adjust the eye-piece, that, on looking through the hole in S', the point P on S
and the reflexion of L in
S' (or really the many
reflexions of P and L)
fall on the same spot,
then the two axes are
not only parallel but
coincident.

The simplest eye-
piece that can be em-
ployed, is a mirror
whose plane coincides
with the axis, and I
adopted this device in
the initial form of my
apparatus. But one-half
of the field of vision is

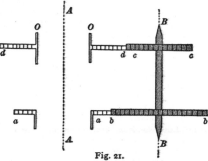

Fig. 21.

lost by this method. A prism of total reflexion, therefore, is much more advantageous. Let ABC (Fig. 22) represent a plane section of such a prismatic

sensations exist, which proceed from this apparatus as from a sense-organ, we may assume that this organ simply disengages innervations after the manner of *reflexes*. Innervation may be voluntary and conscious or involuntary and unconscious. The two different organs from which these proceed may be designated by the letters *WI* and *UI*. Both sorts of innervation

eye-piece cut perpendicularly to the planes of the hypothenuse and the two sides. Let this section include, also, the axis of rotation *ONPQ*, which is parallel to *AB*. The ray which passes along the axis *QP* must, after refrac-

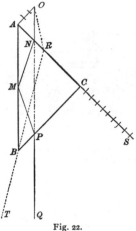

tion and reflexion in the prism, proceed again along the axis *NO* and will meet the eye *O* in the prolongation of the axis. This done, the points of the axis can suffer no displacement from rotation, and the apparatus is centred. The ray in question must accordingly fall at *M*, the middle point of *AB*, and, hence, since it falls on crown glass at an angle of incidence of 45°, will meet *AB* at about 16° 40′. Therefore, *OP* must be distant about 0·115 *AB* from the axis,—a relation which can best be obtained by trial, by so moving the prism in the eye-piece that oscillations of the objects in *gg* during rotation are eliminated.

Fig. 22 also shows the field of vision for the eye at *O*. The ray *OA*, which falls vertically upon *AC*, is reflected at *AB* in the direction *AC* and passes out towards *S*. The ray *OR*, on the other hand, is reflected at *B* and emerges, after refraction, in the direction of *T*.

Fig. 22.

The apparatus has hitherto proved quite sufficient for my experiments. If a printed page is placed in *gg*, and the apparatus turned so rapidly that the image on the retina is entirely obliterated, one can easily read the print through the eye-piece. The inversion of the image by reflexion could be removed by placing a second, stationary reflecting prism above the revolving prism of the eye-piece. But this complication appeared to me unnecessary.

With the exception of a few physical experiments, I have hitherto undertaken rotation-experiments only with various small vertebrates (birds, fishes), and have found the data given in my work on *Motor Sensations* fully confirmed. However, it would probably be of advantage to make similar experiments with insects and other lower animals, especially with marine animals.

may pass to the oculo-motor apparatus (*OM*) and to the locomotor apparatus (*LM*).

Let us now consider the accompanying diagram. We induce by the will, that is by a stimulus from *WI*, an active movement, which passes in the direction of the unfeathered arrows, to *OM* and *LM*. The appurtenant innervation is directly felt. In this case, therefore, a special sensation of movement, differing from the innervation, is unnecessary. If the motion in the direction of the unfeathered arrows is a passive one (taking us by surprise), then, as experience shows, reflexes proceed from *TO* over *UI*, which produce compensatory movements, indicated by the feathered

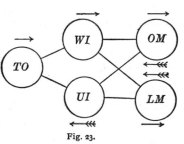

Fig. 23.

arrows. If *WI* takes no part in the process, and the compensation is effected, both the motion and the necessity for motor sensation cease. But if the compensatory movement is intentionally suppressed, that is, by intervention from *WI*, then the same innervation is necessary for achieving this result as for active movement, and it consequently produces the same motor sensation.

The terminal organ *TO* is accordingly so adjusted to *WI* and *UI* that upon a given motor stimulus in the first, contrary innervations are set up in the last

two. But further, we have to notice the following difference in the relation of *TO* to *WI* and *UI*. For
TO, the motor excitation is naturally the same whether
the movement induced is passive or active. In active
movements, too, the innervations proceeding from *WI*
would eventually be neutralised by *TO* and *UI*, did not
inhibitory innervations proceed simultaneously with
the willed innervations from *WI* to *TO* and *UI*. The
influence of *TO* upon *WI* must be conceived as much
weaker than that of *TO* upon *UI*. If we should picture
to ourselves three animals, *WI*, *UI*, and *TO*, between
whom there was a division of labor, such that the first
executed only movements of attack, the second only
those of defence or flight, while the third filled the
post of sentinel, all of whom were united into a single
new organism in which *WI* held the dominant position,
we should have a conception approximately corresponding to the relation represented. There is much
in favor of such a conception of the higher animals.[1]

I do not offer the preceding view as a complete and
perfectly apposite picture of the facts. On the contrary, I am fully aware of the defects in my treatment.

[1] If I grasp a little bird in my hand, the bird will behave towards my hand
exactly as a human being would towards a giant cuttle-fish.—In watching a
company of little children whose movements are largely unreflecting and unpractised, the hands and eyes remind one very strongly of polyphoid creatures. Of course, such impressions do not afford solutions of scientific questions, but it is often very suggestive to abandon oneself to their influence.

[A welcome confirmation of my conjecture of 1875 regarding the *macula
acustica* has been furnished by the subsequent works of Breuer and Kreidl.
The latter has succeeded in causing certain specimens of the Crustacea to
substitute ferrum limatum for their natural otoliths, and they have then re-
acted on magnets by changes of position.—MACH, 1896.]

But the attempt to reduce to a quality of sensation, in accordance with the cardinal principle evolved in our investigation (p. 28), all sensations of space and movement arising in the province of sight and touch during change of place, or even as a shadow in remembrance of locomotion, or at the thought of a distant spot, etc., will be found justifiable. The assumption that this quality of sensation is the will, so far as the latter is occupied with position in space and spatial relation, or the sensation of innervation, does not forestall future investigation and only represents the facts as they are known at the present time.[1]

11.

From the discussions of the previous chapter relative to symmetry and similarity, we may immediately draw the conclusion that to *like* directions of lines which are seen, the same kind of innervation-sensations, and to lines symmetrical with respect to the median plane very *similar* sensations of innervation correspond, but that with looking upwards and looking downwards, or with looking at objects afar off and at the objects near at hand, very *different* sensations of innervation are associated,—as we should naturally be led to expect from the symmetrical arrangement of the motor apparatus of the eye. With this single perception we dispose of a long chain of peculiar physiologico-optical phenomena, which have as yet received

[1] Compare Hering's opinion given in Hermann's *Handbuch der Physiologie*, Vol. III., Part I., p. 547.

scarcely any attention. I now come to the point which, physically regarded at least, is the most important.

The space of the geometrician is a mental construct of threefold manifoldness, that has grown up on the basis of manual and intellectual operations. Optical space (Hering's "sight-space") bears a somewhat complicated geometrical relationship to the former. The matter may be best expressed in familiar terms by saying that optical space represents geometrical space (Euclid's space) in a sort of *relievo-perspective*—a relation of things which may be teleologically explained. In any event, optical space also is a threefold manifoldness. The space of the geometrician exhibits at every point and in all directions the same properties— a quality which is by no means characteristic of physiological space. But the influence of physiological space may nevertheless be abundantly observed in geometry. Such is the case, for example, when we distinguish between convex and concave curvatures. The geometrician should really know only the amount of deviation from the mean of the ordinates.

12.

As long as we conceive the (12) muscles of the eye to be separately innervated, we are not in a position to explain this fundamental fact. I felt this difficulty for years, and also recognised the direction in which, on the principle of the parallelism of the physical and the psychical, the explanation was to be sought ; but owing to my defective experience in this province, the solution itself remained hidden from me. All the better, therefore, am I able to appreciate the service rendered by Hering, who discovered it. To the *three* optical space co-ordinates, viz., to the sensations of height, breadth, and depth, corresponds according to the showing of this investigator (Hering, *Beiträge zur Physiologie,·* Leipsic, Engelmann, 1861–1865) simply a *threefold* innervation, which turns the eyes to the right or to the left, raises or lowers them, and causes them to converge, according to the respective needs of the case. This is the point which I regard as the most important and essential.[1] Whether we regard the innervation itself as the space-sensation, or whether we conceive the space-sensation as ulterior to the innervation,—a question neither easy nor necessary to decide,—nevertheless Hering's statement throws a flood of light on the psychical obscurity of the visual process. The phenomena cited by myself with regard to symmetry and similarity, moreover, accord excellently with this conception. But it is unnecessary, I think, to substantiate further their agreement.[2]

[1] This is the point to which reference was made above (p. 57 and page 68).

[2] This conception also removes a difficulty which I still felt in 1871, and to which I gave utterance in my lecture on "Symmetry" (Prague: Calve 1872),—now translated into English in my *Popular Scientific Lectures*, Chicago, 1894,—in the following words: "The possession of a sense for symmetry by persons who are one-eyed from birth is certainly an enigma. Yet the sense for symmetry, although originally acquired by the eyes, could not have been confined exclusively to the visual organs. By thousands of years of practice it must also have been implanted in other parts of the human organism, and cannot, therefore, be immediately eliminated on the loss of an eye." As a fact, *the symmetrical apparatus of innervation* remains, even when one eye is lost.

THE SIGHT-SENSATIONS.

THEIR RELATIONS TO ONE ANOTHER AND TO
OTHER PSYCHICAL ELEMENTS.

I.

IN normal psychical life, sight-sensations do not make their appearance alone, but are accompanied by other sensations. We do not see *optical* images in an optical space, but we perceive the *bodies* round about us in their many and varied sensuous qualities. Deliberate analysis is needed to single out the sight-sensations from these complexes. Even the total perceptions themselves are almost invariably accompanied by thoughts, wishes, and impulses. By sensations are excited, in animals, the movements of adaptation demanded by their conditions of life. If these conditions are simple, altering but little and slowly, immediate sensory excitation is sufficient.[1]

---

[1] Bearing this circumstance in mind, will prevent our overestimating the intelligence of lower species.

[When the above lines were written, over ten years ago, I had only a few experiences of my own at command. I knew that certain beetles crept only *upwards* on stalks, no matter how often they were turned round, that when they arrived at the top they again invariably flew upwards; that moths always

Higher intellectual development is unnecessary. But the case is different where the conditions of life are intricate and variable. Here so simple a mechanism of adaptation can neither develop, nor would it lead to the accomplishment of the required ends.

Lower species devour everything that comes in their way and that excites the proper stimulus. A more highly developed animal must seek its food at risks to itself; when found, must seize it at the right spot, or capture it by cunning, and cautiously test its character. Long trains of varied memories must pass before its mind before one is sufficiently strong to out-weigh the antagonistic considerations and to excite the appropriate movement. Here, therefore, a sum of associated remembrances (or experiences) coincidently determining the adaptive movements, accompany and confront the sensations. In this consists the intellect.

In the young of higher animals, presenting com-plex conditions of life, the complexes of *sensations* nec-essary to excite adaptive movements are frequently of a very complicated nature.[1] With the development of intelligence, the parts of these complexes necessary

flew towards the light; in short, that certain animals often acted under certain circumstances like automata. Since then much light has been thrown on this subject, and by none more than by the beautiful researches of J. Loeb on *Geotropismus* and *Heliotropismus*. Arrogant underestimation of the intelli-gence of animals has frequently alternated with irrational overestimation of their powers. I regard it as a great service on Sir John Lubbock's part to have paved the way, by his experiments on bees and ants, for more correct ideas on this subject. I also accept here in all essential points the views of C. Lloyd Morgan.—MACH, 1895.]

[1] The sucking of young mammals, and the conduct of the young sparrow described in the note on page 37 are good examples of this.

to produce the excitation constantly diminish, and the sensations are more and more supplemented and replaced by the intellect, as may be daily observed in children and adolescent animals.

2.

Representation by images and ideas, therefore, has to supply the place of sensations, where the latter are imperfect, and to carry to their issue processes initially determined by sensations alone.   But in normal life, representation cannot *supplant* sensation, where this is at all present, except with the greatest danger to the organism.   As a fact, there is, in normal psychical life, a marked difference between the two species of psychical factors.   I see a blackboard before me.   I can, with the greatest vividness, represent to myself on this blackboard, either a hexagon drawn in clear, white lines, or a colored figure.   But, pathological cases apart, I always distinguish what I *see* and what I *represent to myself.*   In the transition to representation, I am aware that my attention is turned from my eyes, and directed elsewhere.   In consequence of this attention, the spot seen upon the blackboard and the one represented to myself as situated in the same place differ as by a fourth co-ordinate.   It would not be a complete description of the facts to say that the representation overlays the object as the images reflected in a transparent plate of glass overlay the bodies seen through it.   We are confronted here, for the time being, with a fundamental psychological fact, the physiological explanation of which will sometime undoubtedly be discovered.

Where the development of intelligence has reached a high point, such as is presented now in the complex conditions of human life, representation may frequently absorb the whole of attention, so that events in the neighborhood of the reflecting person are not noticed, and questions addressed to him are not heard; —a state which persons unused to it are wont to call absent-mindedness, although it might with more appropriateness be called present-mindedness. If the person in question is disturbed in such a state, he has a very distinct sensation of the labor involved in the transference of his attention.

3.

It is well to note this sharp division between representations and sensations, as it is an excellent safeguard against carelessness in psychological explanations of sense-phenomena. The well-known theory of "unconscious reasoning" would never have reached its present extended development if more heed had been paid to this circumstance.

The organ of representation can for the nonce be conceived as one which, in a diminished degree, is susceptible of all the specific energies of the sense and motor organs, so that, according to the special attention evoked, now this, now that specific energy

is excited in it. Such an organ is eminently qualified
for *physiological mediation* between the different energies. As is shown by experiments with animals
whose cerebrum has been removed, there are probably, in addition to the organ of representation, a
number of other, analogous organs of mediation, whose
processes are unconscious.

That wealth of representative life with which we are
personally acquainted from self-observation, doubtless
made its first appearance with man. But the *begin-
nings* of this expression of life, in which nothing but
the relations of the various parts of the organism to
one another is manifested, go back with no less certainty to quite primitive stages in the animal scale.
On the other hand, the parts of single organs must also,
by mutual adaptation, sustain a reciprocal relation to
one another analogous to that of the parts of the organism as a whole. The two retinas, with their motor
mechanism of accommodation and of luminous adjustment, controlled by light sensations, afford a very
clear and familiar example of such a relation. Physiological experiment and simple self-observation teach
us that such an organ has its own adaptive habits, its
own peculiar memory, one might almost say its own
intelligence.

The most instructive observations in this connex·
ion are probably those of Johannes Müller, collected
in his excellent work on "The Phantasms of Sight"
(*Ueber die phantastischen Gesichtserscheinungen.* Cob-

lenz, 1826). The sight-phantasms observed by Müller and others in the waking state are entirely without the control of either the will or the reason. They are independent phenomena, connected not with the organ of representation, but with the sense-organs, and have thoroughly the character of processes objectively seen. They are veritable imagination and memory phenomena of sense.

Those processes which (according to Müller) are normally induced in the visual substance by excitations of the retina, and which condition the act of seeing, may also, under certain conditions, be spontaneously produced in the visual substance without excitation of the retina, becoming there the source of phantasms or hallucinations. We speak of *sense-memory* when the phantasms are closely allied in character to objects seen before, of *hallucinations* when the phantoms arise more freely and independently. But no sharp distinction between the two cases can be maintained.[1]

[1] I am acquainted with all manner of sight-phantasms from my own experience. The mingling of phantasms with objects indistinctly seen, the latter being partly supplanted, are probably the most common. Years ago, while engrossed with the study of pulse-tracings and sphygmography, the fine white curves on the dark background often came up before my eyes, in the evening or in the dim light of day, with the full semblance of reality and objectivity. Later also, during work in physics, I witnessed analogous phenomena of "sense-memory." More rarely, images of things which I have never seen before, have appeared before my eyes in the day-time. Thus, years ago, on a number of successive days, a bright red capillary net (similar to a so-called enchanted net) shone out upon the book in which I was reading, or on my writing paper, although I had never been occupied with forms of this sort. The sight of bright-colored changing carpet patterns before falling asleep was very familiar to me in my youth; the phenomenon will still make its appearance if I fix my attention on it. One of my children, likewise, often tells

When we withdraw the retina from the influence of outward excitations, and turn the attention to the field of vision alone, traces of phantasms are almost always present. Indeed, they make their appearance when the outer excitations are merely weak and indistinct, in a poor and dull light, or when we look, for example, at a surface covered with dim, blurred spots, or at a cloud, or at a grey wall. The figures which we then seem to see, provided they are not produced by a direct act of attention in selecting and combining distinctly visible spots, are certainly not products of representation, but constitute, at least in part, spontaneous phantasms, which, for the time being and at some points, take forcible precedence over the retinal excitation.[1]

me of "seeing flowers" before falling asleep. Less often, I see in the evening, before falling asleep, manifold human figures, which alter without the action of my will. On a single occasion I attempted successfully to change a human face into a fleshless skull; this solitary instance may, however, be an accident. It has often happened to me that, on awaking in a dark room, the images of my latest dreams remained present in vivid colors and in abundant light. A peculiar phenomenon, which has for some years frequently occurred with me is the following. I awake and lie motionless with my eyes closed. Before me I see the bedspread with all its little folds, and upon the latter, motionless and unchanging, my hands in all their details. If I open my eyes, either it is quite dark, or it is light, but the spread and my hands lie quite differently from the manner in which they appeared to me. This a remarkably fixed and persistent phantasm with me, such as I have not observed under other conditions.

1 Leonardo da Vinci discusses the mingling of phantasms with objects seen, *loc. cit.*, p. 56, in the following words:

"I shall not omit to give a place among these directions to a newly dis-
"covered sort of observation, which may, indeed, make a small and almost
"ludicrous appearance, but which is, nevertheless, very useful in awakening
"the mind to various discoveries. It consists in this, that thou shouldst re-
"gard various walls which are covered with all manner of spots, or stone of
"different composition. If thou hast any capacity for discovery, thou mayest
"behold there things which resemble various landscapes decked with moun-

All marked and independent appearance of phantasms without excitation of the retina—dreams and the half-waking state excepted—must, by reason of their biological purposelessness, be accounted pathological. In like manner, we are constrained to regard every abnormal dependence of phantasms upon the *will* as pathological. Such, very likely, are the states that occur in insane persons who regard themselves as very powerful, as God, etc.

4.

After these introductory considerations we may now turn to the consideration of a few physiologico-optical phenomena, the full explanation of which, it is true, is still distant, but which are best understood as the expressions of an *independent life* on the part of the sense-organs.

"tains, rivers, cliffs, trees, large plains, hills and valleys of many a sort. Thou "canst also behold all manner of battles, life-like positions of strange, un- "familiar figures, expressions of face, costumes, and numberless things "which thou mayest put into good and perfect form. The experience with "regard to walls and stone of this sort is similar to that of the ringing of "bells, in the strokes of which thou willst find anew every name and every "word that thou mayest imagine to thyself.

 "Do not despise this opinion of mine when I counsel thee sometimes to "pause and look at the spots on walls, or the ashes in the fire, or the clouds, "or mud, or other places; thou willst make very wonderful discoveries in "them, if thou observest them rightly. For the mind of the painter is stim- "ulated by them to many new discoveries, be it in the composition of battles, "of animals and human beings, or in various compositions of landscapes, "and of monstrous things, as devils and the like, which are calculated to "bring thee honor. That is, through confused and undefined things the mind "is awakened to new discoveries. But take heed, first, that thou understand- "est how to shape well all the members of the things that thou wishest to "represent, for instance, the limbs of living beings, as also the parts of a "landscape, namely the stones, trees, and the like."

We usually see with both eyes, and agreeably to definite needs of life, not colors and forms, but bodies in space. Not the elements of the complex, but the physiologico-optical complex *entire*, is of importance. This complex the eye seeks to fill out and supplement, according to the habits acquired (or inherited) under its environment, whenever, as a result of special circumstances, the appearance of the complex is incomplete. This occurs oftenest in monocular vision, but is also possible in the binocular observation of very distant objects where the stereoscopic differences consequent upon the distance of the eyes from each other vanish.

We generally perceive, not light and shadow, but objects in space. The shading of bodies is scarcely noticed. Differences of illumination produce differences in the sensation of depth, and help to define the form of bodies where the stereoscopic differences are insufficient,—a condition which is very noticeable in the observation of distant mountains.

Very instructive, in this relation, is the image on the dull plate of the photographic camera. We are often astounded at the brightness of the lights and the depth of the shadows, which were not noticed in the bodies themselves but are striking when brought into a *single* plane. I remember quite well that, in my childhood, all shading appeared to me an unjustifiable disfigurement of drawing, and that an outline-sketch was much more satisfactory to me. It is likewise well-known that whole peoples, for instance the Chinese, despite a well-developed artistic technique, do not shade at all, or shade only in a defective manner.

The following experiment, which I made many years ago, illustrates very clearly the above-noticed relation between light-sensation and the sensation of depth. We place a visiting-card, bent cross-wise, before us on the desk, so that its bent edge is towards us. Let the light fall from the left. The half *a b d e* is then much lighter, the half *b c e f* much darker—a fact which is, however, scarcely perceived in unprejudiced observation. We now close one eye. Hereupon, part of the space-sensations disappear. Still we see the bent card in space and nothing noticeable in the illumination. But as  soon as we succeed in seeing the bent edge depressed instead of raised, the light and the shade stand out as if painted thereon. Such an inversion is possible, because depth is not determined in monocular vision.

Fig. 24.

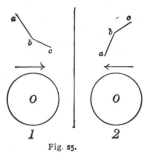

Fig. 25.

If in Fig. 25, 1 *O* represents the eye, *a b c* a section of a bent card, and the arrow the direction of the light, *a b* will appear lighter than *b c*. Also in 2, *a b* will appear lighter than *b c*. Plainly, the eye must acquire the habit of interchanging the illumination of the sur-

face-elements and the fall of the depth-sensation. The
fall and the depth diminish, with diminishing illumination, towards the right, when the light falls from the
left (1); contrariwise, when it falls from the right.
Since the wrappings of the ball in which the retina is
embedded are translucent, it is not a matter of indiffer-
ence for the distribution of light upon the retina
whether the light falls from the right or the left.   Accordingly, things are so arranged that,* without any
aid of judgment, a fixed habit of the eye is developed,
by means of which illumination and depth are definitely connected. If, by virtue of another habit then,
it is possible to bring a part of the retina into conflict
with the first habit, as in the above experiment, the
effect is made manifest by remarkable sensations.

The purpose of the preceding remarks is merely to
point out the character of the phenomenon under consideration and to indicate the direction in which a
physiological explanation (exclusive of psychological
speculation) is to be sought. We will further remark
that, with respect to interchangeable qualities of sensation, a principle similar to that of the conservation
of energy seems to hold. Differences of illumination
are partly transformed into differences of perspective
depth, and in this transformation are weakened in their
first capacity. At the expense of differences of depth,
on the other hand, differences of illumination may be
augmented. An analogous observation will be made
later on in another connexion.

5.

The habit of observing *bodies* as such, that is, of giving attention to a large and spatially cohering mass of light-sensations, carries within it a source of peculiar and ever astonishing phenomena. A two-colored painting or drawing, for instance, appears in general quite different according as we take the one or the other color as the background. The puzzle pictures, in which, for example, an apparition makes its appearance between tree-trunks as soon as the dark trees are taken as the background, and the bright sky as the object, are well known. In exceptional instances only do background and object possess the same form— a configuration frequently employed in ornamental designs, as may be seen in

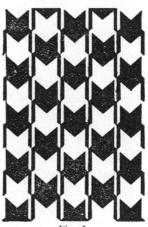

Fig. 26.

Fig. 26, taken from page 15 of the afore-mentioned *Grammar of Ornament*, also in Figs. 20 and 22 of Plate 35, and in Fig. 13 of Plate 43 of that work.

6.

The phenomena of space-vision which accompany the monocular observation of a perspective drawing, or, what amounts to the same thing, the monocular observation of a spatial object, are generally very lightly passed over, as being self-evident in nature. But I am of the opinion that there is yet much to be investigated in these phenomena. One and the same perspective drawing may represent an unlimited number of different objects, and consequently the space-sensation can be only *in part* determined by such a drawing. If, therefore, despite the many bodies conceivable as belonging to the figure, only a few are really seen with the full character of objectivity, there must exist some good reason for the coincidence. It cannot arise from the adducing of auxiliary considerations in *thought*, nor from the awakening of conscious remembrances in any form, but must depend on certain *organic habitudes* of the visual sense.

If the visual sense acts in conformity with the habits which it has acquired through adaptation to the life-conditions of the species and the individual, we may, in the first place, assume that it proceeds according to the principle of Probability ; that is, those functions which have been most frequently excited together before, will afterwards tend to make their appearance together when only one is excited. For example, those particular sensations of depth which in the past have been most frequently associated with a given perspective figure, will be extremely likely to reproduce themselves again when that figure makes its appearance, although not necessarily *co-determined* thereby. Furthermore, a principle of economy appears to manifest itself in the observation of perspective drawings; that is to say, the visual sense never of itself puts forth greater efforts than are demanded by the excitation. The two principles coincide in their results, as we shall presently see.

7.

The following may serve as a detailed illustration of the above. When we look at a straight line in a perspective drawing, we always see it as a straight line in space, although the straight line as a perspective drawing may correspond to an unlimited number of different plane spatial curves. But only in the special case where the plane of a curve passes through the centre of one eye, will it be delineated on the retina in question as a straight line (or as a great circle), and only in the yet more special case where the plane of the curve passes through the centres of both eyes, will it be delineated on both as a straight line. It is thus extremely improbable that a plane curve should ever appear a straight line, while on the other hand a straight line in space is always reflected upon both retinas as a straight line. The most probable object, therefore, answering to a perspective straight line, is a spatial straight line.

The straight line has various *geometrical* properties. But these geometrical properties, for example the

familiar characteristic of being the shortest distance between two points, are not *physiologically* of importance.
It is of far more consequence that straight lines lying
in the median plane or perpendicular thereto are physiologically symmetrical to themselves. A vertical
lying in the median plane is also physiologically distinguished by its perfect uniformity of depth-sensation, and by its coincidence with the direction of gravity. All vertical straight lines may be readily and
quickly made to coincide with the median plane, and
consequently partake of this physiological advantage.
But the spatial straight line *generally*, must be physiologically distinguished by some different mark. Its
sameness of *direction* in all its elements has already
been pointed out. In addition to this, however, it is
to be noted that every point of a straight line in space
marks the *mean* of the depth-sensations of the neighboring points. Thus the straight line in space represents a *minimum of departure from the mean of the depth-
sensations* ; and the assumption forthwith presents
itself that the straight line is seen *with the least effort*.
The visual sense acts therefore in conformity with the
principle of economy, and, at the same time, in conformity with the principle of probability, when it exhibits a preference for straight lines.[1]

[1] As early as 1866, I wrote, in the *Proceedings of the Vienna Academy*, Vol.
54: "Since straight lines everywhere surround civilised human beings, we
may, I think, assume, that every straight line which can possibly be produced
upon the retina has been seen numberless times, in every possible way, spatially as a straight line. The efficiency of the eye in the interpretation of
straight lines ought not, therefore, to astonish us." Even then I wrote this

8.

The deviation of a sensation from the mean of the adjacent sensations is always noticeable, and exacts a special effort on the part of the sense-organ. Every new turn of a curve, every projection or depression of a surface, involves a deviation of some space-sensation from the mean of the surrounding field on which the attention is directed. The plane is distinguished physiologically by the fact that this deviation from the mean is a minimum, or for each point in particular $= 0$. In looking through a stereoscope at a spotted surface, the separate images of which have not yet been combined into a binocular view, we experience a peculiarly agreeable impression when the whole is suddenly flattened out into a plane. The æsthetic impressions produced by the circle and the sphere seem to have their source mainly in the fact that the above-mentioned deviation from the mean is the same for all points.

That the deviation from the mean of adjacent parts plays a rôle in light-sensation I pointed out many years ago.[1] If a row of black and white sectors, such

passage (opposing the Darwinian view, which I supported in the same paper) half-heartedly. To-day I am more than ever convinced that the efficiency referred to is not the result of individual functioning, nor indeed of human functioning, but that it is also characteristic of animals, and is, at least in part, a matter of inheritance.

[1] "Ueber die Wirkung der räumlichen Vertheilung des Lichtreizes auf die Netzhaut." *Sitzungsberichte der Wiener Akademie* (1865), Vol. 52. Continuation of the same inquiry: *Sitzber.* (1866), Vol. 54; *Sitzber.* (1868), Vol. 57; *Vierteljahrsschrift für Psychiatrie*, Neuwied-Leipzig, 1868, (" Ueber die Abhängigkeit der Netzhautstellen von einander ").

as are shown in Fig. 27, be painted on a strip of
paper *A A BB*, and this be then wrapped about a cylinder the axis of which is parallel to *AB*, there will be
produced, on the rapid rotation of the latter, a grey
field with increasing illumination from *B* to *A*, in
which, however, a bright line *α α*, and a dark line
β β, make their appearance. The points which correspond to the indentations *α* are not physically brighter
than the neighboring parts, but their light-intensity

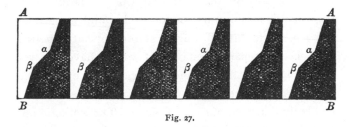

Fig. 27.

exceeds the mean intensity of the immediately adjacent parts, while, on the other hand, the light-intensity
at *β* falls short of the mean intensity of the adjacent
parts.[1] This deviation from the mean is distinctly
felt, and accordingly imposes a special burden upon
the organ of sight.   Of what significance this circumstance is for saliency and the sharp spatial definition
of objects, I pointed out long ago.

[1] A remark concerning the analogies between light-sensation and the potential function will be found in my note "Concerning Mr. Guébhard's Representation of Equipotential Curves," *Wiedemann's Annalen* (1882), Vol.
XVII., p. 864.

9.

With regard to the depth-sensation excited by a drawing viewed monocularly, the following experiments are instructive. Fig. 28 is a plane quadrilateral with its two diagonals. If we regard it monocularly, it is most easily seen, according to the law of probability, as a plane. In the great majority of cases, objects which are not plane, *force* the eye to the vision of depth. Where this compulsion is lacking, the plane object is the most probable and at the same time the easiest for the organ of sight.

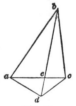

Fig. 28.

The same drawing may be also viewed monocularly as a tetrahedron, the edge *b d* of which lies in front of *a c*, or as a tetrahedron, the edge *b d* of which lies back of *a c*. The influence of the imagination and the will upon the visual process is extremely limited; it is restricted to the directing of the attention and to the *selection* of the appropriate *disposition* of the organ of sight for one of a number of cases given by habit, of which, however, each one, when chosen, runs its course with mechanical certainty and precision. Looking at the point *e*, we can, as a fact, produce either of the two optically possible tetrahedrons at will, according as we represent to ourselves *b d* nearer or farther away than *a c*. The organ of sight is practised in the representation of these two cases, since it often happens that one body is partly concealed by another.

The same figure may, finally, be seen as a four-sided pyramid, if we imagine the conspicuously situated point of intersection *e* before or behind the plane *a b c d*. This is difficult to do, if *b e d* and *a e c* are two perfectly straight lines, because it conflicts with the habit of the organ of sight to see, without constraint, a straight line bent ; the effort is successful only because the point *e* has a conspicuous position. But if there is a slight indentation at *e*, the attempt involves no difficulty.

The effect of a linear perspective drawing is felt as unerringly by one who is ignorant of perspective as by one who is thoroughly conversant with the theory, provided the former is able to disregard the plane of the drawing,—a condition readily fulfilled in monocular observation. Reflexion, and even the remembrance of seen objects, have, according to my belief, little or nothing to do with the effect in question. Why the straight lines of a drawing are seen as spatial straight lines, has already been pointed out. Where straight lines appear to converge to a point in the plane of the drawing, the converging or approaching ends are referred, according to the principle of probability and economy, to like or to nearly like depth. Herewith we have the effect of the vanishing points. Such lines may be seen parallel, but there is no necessity for such an impression. If we hold the drawing, Fig. 29, on a level with the eye, it may represent to us a glance down a passage-way. The ends *g h e f* are referred to like distances. If the distance is great, the lines *a e, b f, c g, d h* appear horizontal. If we raise the drawing, the ends *e f g h* rise, and the floor *a b e f* seems to have an upward slope.

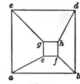

Upon lowering the drawing, the opposite phenomenon is presented; and analogous changes may be observed by moving the drawing towards the right or the left. In these facts, the

Fig. 29.

elements of perspective effect find simple and clear expression.

Plane drawings, provided they consist entirely of straight lines, everywhere intersecting each other at right angles, almost always appear plane. If oblique intersections and curved lines occur, the lines easily pass out of the plane; as is shown, for example, by Fig. 30, which may, without difficulty, be conceived as a curved sheet of paper. When outlines, such as are represented in Fig. 30, have assumed definite spatial form, and are seen as the

Fig. 30.

boundary of a surface, the latter, to describe it briefly, appears *as flat as possible*, that is to say, is presented with a minimum of deviation from the mean of the depth-sensation.[1]

_____

[1] Here again, the depth-sensation resembles the potential function, in a space at the boundaries of which it is determined. This flat-as-possible sur

10.

The peculiar action of lines intersecting obliquely in the plane of the drawing (or on the retina), whereby the same are mutually and jointly forced out of the plane of the drawing (or out of the plane perpendicu-

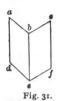

Fig. 31.

lar to the line of sight) was first observed by me on the occasion of the above-mentioned (p. 91) experiment with the monocular inversion of a card. The card in Fig. 31, whose edge *be* when turned outwards is in a vertical position, assumes, on my seeing *be* depressed, a recumbent position, like that of a book lying open upon my table, with the result that *b* appears *farther away* than *e*. When one is perfectly acquainted with the phenomenon, the inversion may

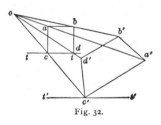

Fig. 32.

be performed with almost every object, and one can always observe along with the change of *form* (along with the flapping) a remarkable simultaneous change of *position*. The effect is especially astonishing in the case of transparent objects. Let *a b c d* be a section of a glass cube lying on a table *t t*, and let *O* be the eye. (Fig. 32.) On monocular inversion, the angle *a* is projected to *a'*,

face does not coincide with the surface of minimal area, which would be obtained if the spatial outlines were made of wire, and then dipped in soapsuds, producing a liquid film of Plateau.

b to the nearer point *b'*, *c* to *c'*, and *d* to *d'*. The cube will seem to stand obliquely on its edge *c'* upon the table *t' t'*. In order that the drawing might afford a better survey of the phenomenon, the two views have been represented behind, not within one another. If a drinking-glass partly filled with a colored liquid be substituted for the cube, it will be seen, together with the surface of the liquid, in a similar oblique position.

With sufficient attention, the same phenomena may be provoked in any linear drawing. If we place the page containing Fig. 31 vertically before us, and observe it monocularly, we shall see *b* project if *b e* be raised, but if *b e* be depressed *b* will retreat and *e* will project and come nearer to the observer. It may be said, briefly, that the legs of *acute* angles are thrust out on *different* sides of the plane of the drawing, or of the plane perpendicular to the line of sight, but that the legs of *obtuse* angles are thrust out on the *same* side. We may also say that all angles exhibit the tendency to become *right* angles.

I was not long in discovering that the phenomenon referred to differed in no essential respect from that presented by Zöllner's pseudoscopy. Although these phenomena have been much studied, no satisfactory explanation of them has as yet been offered. Naturally such superficial explanations as, for instance, the assumption that we are chiefly accustomed to see *right* angles, are inadmissible, if the investigation is not utterly to miscarry or to be prematurely broken off. We see oblique-angled objects often enough, but never, without artificial preparation, the motionless, oblique surface of a liquid, as we did in the experiment given above. Yet, the eye, it would seem, prefers the oblique liquid surface to an oblique-angled body.

11.

The elemental power displayed in these processes has, I believe, its root in far simpler habits of the organ of sight,—habits whose origin doubtless antedates the civilised life of man. I have essayed to explain the phenomena in question by a contrast of directions analogous to the contrast of colors, but without arriving at a satisfactory result. The principle of economy likewise affords me no enlightenment.

A somewhat greater prospect of success seems to be offered by the principle of probability. Let us conceive the retina as a perfect sphere and imagine the eye fixed upon the vertex of an angle a in space. The planes passing through the centre of the eye and the lines containing the angle, project the latter upon the retina, describing thereon a spherical segment having the angle A, which represents the angle of the monocular *image.* An infinite number of values for a, now, varying from $0°$ to $180°$, may correspond to a constant value of A, as will be seen if we reflect that the lines including the objective angle may assume every possible position in the planes yielding their projections.

Consequently, to a *seen* angle *A* we may have corresponding, all the possible values of the objective angle *a* that can be obtained by causing each of the sides, *b* and *c*, of the triangle to vary between 0° and 180°. The result is, supposing the calculation to be performed in a definite manner, that *larger* angles are the most probable objects corresponding to observed *acute* angles, and *smaller* angles the most likely counterparts of observed *obtuse* angles. I was not, however, in a position to determine whether the phenomena in question, which we might be inclined to regard as *geometrically* alike, could also be regarded as *physiologically* the same—a question which is both essential and important. Moreover, the whole conception has still a slightly too artificial cast for me.

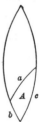

Fig. 33.

12.

A plane linear drawing, monocularly observed, frequently appears plane. But if the angles be made to vary and motion be introduced, every drawing of this sort will assume a solid form. We generally see, then, a solid body in rotation, such as I have described on a former occasion.[1] The well-known acoustic figures of Lissajous, which on varying their difference of phase, appear to lie on a revolving cylinder, afford an excellent example of the process in question.

[1] "Beobachtungen über monoculare Stereoscopie," *Sitzungsberichte der Wiener Akademie* (1868), Vol. 58.

Here, again, reference might be made to our habit of constantly dealing with solid bodies. In fact, solid bodies engaged in revolutions and turnings continually surround us. Indeed, the whole material world in which we move is, to a certain extent, a continuous solid body ; and without the help of solid bodies we could never attain to the conception of geometrical space. We do not generally notice the position of the single points of a body in space, but apprehend directly its dimensions. Herein lies, for the unpractised, the main difficulty of drawing a perspective picture. Children, who are accustomed to *seeing* bodies in their real dimensions, do not understand perspective foreshortenings, and are far better satisfied with simple contours, with outline-drawings. I can well remember this condition of mind, and through this remembrance am able to comprehend the drawings of the ancient Egyptians, who represent all parts of the body as far as possible in their true dimensions, thus pressing them, as it were, into the plane of the drawing, as plants are pressed in a herbarium. In the frescoes of the Pompeians, too, we still meet with a perceptible disinclination to foreshortening, although here the sense of perspective is already manifest. The ancient Italians, on the other hand, in the consciousness of their perfect mastery of the subject, often amuse themselves with excessive and sometimes even unbeautiful foreshortenings, which occasionally demand of the eye considerable exertion.

13.

There can be no question, therefore, but the seeing of solid bodies with the distances between their
salient points unchanged is much easier to us through
habit than is the elimination of the marks of solidity,
which is always the result, in the first place, of deliberate analysis. Accordingly, we may expect that
wherever a coherent mass, which from its common
coloring is apprehended as a *unit*, exhibits spatial alteration, the altering process will be seen preferably
as the motion of a *solid* body. I must confess, however, that this conception is little satisfactory to me.
I believe, rather, that here, too, an *elemental* habit of
the organ of sight is at the root of the matter,—a habit
which was not originally acquired by the conscious
experience of the individual, but, on the contrary,
antecedently facilitated our apprehension of the movements of solid bodies. If we should assume, for example, that every *diminution* of the transverse dimension of an optical sensation-mass to which the attention was directed had the tendency to induce a corresponding *augmentation* of the dimension of depth,
and *vice versa*, we should have a process quite analogous to that which we have already considered above
and which was compared to the conservation of energy. This view is certainly much simpler and supplies an adequate explanation. Furthermore, it en-
ables us to comprehend more easily how so elemental

a habit could be acquired, how it could find expression in the organism, and how the tendency for the same could be inherited.

As a sort of counterpart to the rotation of solid bodies exhibited to us by the organ of sight, I will cite here an additional observation. If an egg, or ellipsoid with dull, uniform surface be rolled over the top of a table, but in such manner that it does not turn about its axis of generation, but performs jolting movements, we shall fancy we see, on viewing it binocularly, a liquid body, or large oscillating drop. The phenomenon is still more noticeable if the egg, with its longitudinal axis in a horizontal position, be set in moderately rapid rotation about a vertical axis. This effect is immediately destroyed when marks, whose movements we may follow, are made upon the surface of the egg. A rotating solid body is then seen.

The explanations offered in this chapter are certainly far from complete, yet I believe that the considerations adduced will have some effect in stimulating and preparing the way for a more exact and thorough study of these phenomena.

TIME-SENSATION.[1]

I.

MUCH more difficult than the investigation of space-sensation is that of time-sensation. Many sensations make their appearance with, others without, space-sensation. But time-sensation accompanies every other sensation, and can be wholly separated from none. We are referred, therefore, in our investigations here, to the *variations* of time-sensation. With this psychological difficulty is associated another, consisting of the fact that the physiological processes underlying the time-sensation are less known, more radical, and more thoroughly concealed than the processes underlying the other sensations. Our analysis, therefore, must confine itself chiefly to the psychological side, without approaching the question from its physical aspect, as is possible, in part at least, in the provinces of the other senses.

[1] The position which I here take differs only slightly from that of my "Untersuchungen über den Zeitsinn des Ohres," *Sitzber. d. Wiener Akademie*, Vol. 51, 1865. Into the details of these earlier experiments, begun in 1860, I shall not enter again here.

2.

That a definite, specific time-sensation exists, appears to me beyond all doubt.   The rhythmical identity of the two adjoined measures, which vary utterly

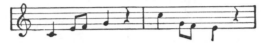

in the order of their tones, is *immediately* recognised. We have not to do here with a matter of the understanding or of reflexion, but with one of sensation. In the same manner that bodies of different colors may possess the same *spatial* form, so here we have two tonal entities which, acoustically, are differently colored, but possess the same *temporal* form.   As in the one case we pick out by an immediate act of feeling the identical spatial components, so here we immediately detect the identical temporal components, or the sameness of the rhythm.

3.

On hearing a number of strokes of a bell, which are exactly alike acoustically, I discriminate between the first, second, third, and so on. Do the accompanying thoughts, perhaps, or other accidental sensations, with which the strokes of the bell happen to be associated, afford these distinguishing marks?   I do not believe that any one will seriously uphold this view. How uncertain and unreliable would our estimate of time prove in such an event! What would become of it if that accidental background of thought and sensation should suddenly vanish from memory ?

While I am reflecting upon something, the clock strikes, but I give no heed to it. After it has finished striking, it may be of importance to me to count the strokes. And as a fact, there arise in my memory distinctly one, two, three, four strokes. I give here my whole attention to this recollection, and by this means the subject on which I was reflecting during the striking of the clock, for the moment completely vanishes from me. The supposed background against which I could note the strokes of the bell, is now wanting to me. By what mark, then, do I distinguish the *second* stroke from the *first ?* Why do I not regard all the strokes, which in other respects are identical, as *one ?* Because each is connected for me with a special time-sensation which starts up into consciousness along with it. In like manner, I distinguish an image present in my memory from a creation of fancy by a specific time-sensation different from that of the present moment.

4.

Since, so long as we are conscious, time-sensation is always present, it is probable that it is connected with the organic *consumption* necessarily associated with consciousness,—that we feel the *work of attention* as time. During severe effort of attention time is long to us, during easy employment short. In phlegmatic conditions, when we scarcely notice our surroundings, the hours pass rapidly away. When our attention is completely exhausted, we sleep. In dreamless sleep, the sensation of time is lacking. When profound sleep intervenes, yesterday is connected with to-day only by an intellectual bond.

The fatiguing of the organ of consciousness goes on continually in waking hours, and the labor of attention increases just as continually. The sensations connected with greater expenditure of attention appear to us to happen *later*.

Normal as well as abnormal psychical acts appear to accord with this conception. Since the attention cannot be fixed upon two different sense-organs at once, the sensations of two organs can never occur together and yet be accompanied by an absolutely equivalent effort of attention. Seemingly, therefore, the one occurs *later* than the other. A parallel of this so-called personal equation of astronomers, having its ground in analogous facts, is also frequently observed in the *same* sense-province. It is a well-known fact that an optical impression which arises physically *later* may yet, under certain circumstances, appear to occur earlier. It sometimes happens, for example, that a surgeon, in bleeding, first sees the blood burst forth and afterwards his lancet enter.[1] Dvorak has shown,[2] in a series of experiments which he carried

[1] Compare Fechner, *Psychophysik*. Leipsic, 1860. Vol. II., p. 433.

[2] Dvorak, "Ueber Analoga der persönlichen Differenz zwischen beiden Augen und den Netzhautstellen desselben Auges." *Sitzber. d. königl. böhm. Gesellschaft der Wissenschaften, (Math.-naturw. Classe)*, vom 8. März, 1872.

out at my desire, years ago, that this relation may be produced at will, the object on which the attention is centred appearing (even in the case of an actual tardiness of 1/8–1/6 of a second) earlier than that indirectly seen. It is quite possible that the familiar experience of the surgeon may find its explanation in this fact. The time which the attention requires to turn from one place at which it is occupied, to another, is shown in the following experiment instituted by me.[1] Two bright red squares measuring two centimetres across and situated on a black background eight centimetres apart, are illuminated in a perfectly dark room by an electric spark concealed from the eye. The square directly seen appears red, but that indirectly seen appears *green,*—and often quite intensely so. The tardy attention finds the indirectly seen square when it is already in the stage of Purkinje's positive after-image. A Geissler's tube with two bright red spots at a short distance from one another, exhibits, on the passage of a single discharge, the same phenomenon.

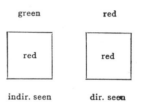

Fig. 34.

5.

The following interesting experience should be cited here. Frequently I have been sitting in my room,

[1] Communicated by Dvorak, *loc. cit.*

absorbed in work, while in an adjacent room experiments in explosions were being carried on. It regularly occurred that I shrank back startled, *before* I heard the report.

Since the attention is especially inert in dreams, naturally the most peculiar anachronisms occur in this state, as every one has doubtless observed. For instance, we dream of a man who rushes at us with a revolver and shoots, awake suddenly, and perceive the object which, by its fall, has produced the entire dream. Now there is nothing absurd in assuming that the acoustic excitation enters simultaneously different nerve-tracks and is met there by the attention in some inverted order, just as, in the case above mentioned, I perceived first the general disturbance of the organism and afterwards the report of the explosion. But in many cases it is undoubtedly sufficient to assume the introduction of sensations into the framework of a dream already present.

6.

If time-sensation is conditioned by progressive organic consumption[1] or by the corresponding steady

---

1 If the consumption, or, for that matter, the accumulation of a "fatigue-material" were *immediately* felt, we might logically expect a reversion of time in dreams. The eccentricities of dreams may *all* be accounted for by the fact that some sensations and representations do not enter consciousness at all, while others enter with too much difficulty and too late. The intellect often sleeps only in part. We converse very sensibly, in dreams, with persons long deceased, but with no recollection of their death. We reflect, in the dream-state, concerning dreams, recognise them as such by their eccentricities, but are immediately pacified again. I once dreamed very vividly of a mill. The water flowed downwards, in a sloping channel, away from the

increase of the effort following upon attention, then it is intelligible why physiological time is *not reversible* but moves only in one direction. As long as we are in the waking state consumption and the labor of attention can only increase, not diminish. The two accompanying bars of music, which present a symmetry to the eye and to the understanding, show nothing of the sort as regards the sensation of time. In the province of rhythm, and of time in general, there is no symmetry.

7.

It is a perfectly natural, though somewhat imperfect conception, to regard the organ of consciousness as capable, in a weakened degree, of *all* the specific energies, of which each sense-organ is capable only of a *few*. Hence the shadowy and evanescent character of representation as compared with sensation, through which it must be constantly nourished and revivified.

mill, and hard by, in just such another channel, upwards to the mill. I was not at all disturbed by the contradiction.—At a time when much engrossed with the subject of space-sensation, I dreamed of a walk in the woods. Suddenly I noticed the defective perspective displacement of the trees, and by this recognised that I was dreaming. The missing displacements, however, were immediately supplied.—Again, while dreaming, I saw in my laboratory a beaker filled with water, in which a candle was serenely burning. "Where does it get its oxygen from?" I thought. "It is absorbed in the water," was the answer. "Where do the gases produced in the combustion go to?" The bubbles from the flame, mounted upwards in the water, and I was satisfied.

[Remarkable observations concerning dreams, which I have frequently verified in my own personal experience, may be found in a book published by W. Robert, entitled *Der Traum als Naturnothwendigkeit* (Hamburg: Hermann Seippel. 1886).—MACH, 1895.]

Hence also the capacity of consciousness to serve as a *bridge of communication* between all sensations and memories. With *every* specific energy of the organ of consciousness, we should then have to conceive still another particular energy, the sensation of time, associated, so that none of the former could be excited without evoking the latter. Should this new energy appear physiologically superfluous and only invented *ad hoc*, we might at once assign to it an important physiological function. What if this energy kept up *the flow of blood* that nourishes the brain-parts in their work, guided this current to its destination, and regulated it? Our conception of attention and of time-sensation would then receive a very material basis. The fact that there is but *one* continuous time, too, would become intelligible, since the partial attention given to one sense is always drawn from the total attention, and is determined by it.

8.

In listening to a number of similar strokes from a bell, we can distinguish each from the others and also count them in memory, provided they are few in number. If the number is large, however, we distinguish the last ones from one another, but not the first. In this case, if we would not make a mistake, we must *count* them immediately upon their being sounded, that is, we must consciously connect with each stroke some ordinal symbol. The phenomenon has a perfect analogue in the province of the space-sense, and is to be explained on the same principle. In walking forwards, we have a distinct sensation that we are moving away from a starting-point, but the *physiological* measure of this removal is not *proportional* to the geometrical. In the same manner, elapsed physiological time is subject to perspective contraction, its single elements becoming less and less distinguishable.[1]

9.

If a special time-sensation exists, it goes without saying that the identity of two rhythms will be immediately recognised. But we must not leave the fact unnoticed that two rhythms which are the same physically may appear very different physiologically, just as the same space-figure by change of position may give rise to different physiological space-forms. The rhythm represented by the following notes, for exam-

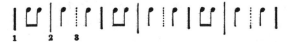

ple, appears quite different according as we regard the short thick, or the long thin vertical lines, or the rows of dots, as the bars. The reason of this is manifestly that the attention (guided by the accent) is *discharged*, so to speak, at 1, 2, or 3, that is, that the sensations of time corresponding to the successive beats are *compared* with different initial sensations.

[1] Compare p. 64.

The rhythm represented in the following diagram appears physiologically similar to the preceding, but only when similarly-marked bars are taken in the two

—that is, when the attention is introduced at homologous points of time.   Two physical time-figures may be termed similar when all the parts of the one stand in the same relation to one another as do the homologous parts of the other.   But physiological similarity makes its appearance only when the above condition is likewise fulfilled.   Furthermore, so far as I am able to judge, we recognise the identity of the time-ratios of two rhythms only when the same are capable of being represented by very small whole numbers.   Thus we really notice immediately, only the identity or non-identity of two times, and, in the latter case, recognise the ratio of the two only by the fact that one part is exactly contained in the other.   Herewith we have an explanation of the fact that, in marking time, the time is always divided into absolutely equal parts.[1]

[1] The similarity of space-figures would be felt, according to this theory, much more immediately than the similarity of rhythms. The connexion between rhythmic movements and the measurement of time, which probably has an important teleological import, need not be discussed here.

SENSATIONS OF TONE.[1]

I.

IN tone-sensations, also, we are restricted mainly to psychological analysis. As before, the initial elements of the investigation are all we can offer.

Among the sensations of tone possessing greatest importance for us are those produced by the human voice, in the form of utterances of pleasure and pain, of expressions of the will, and of the communication of thoughts by speech, etc. The voice and the organ of hearing doubtless bear a close relation to each other. The simplest and distinctest form in which sensations of tone reveal their remarkable characteristics is music. Will, feeling, vocal expression and vocal sense-receptivity have certainly a strong physiological connexion. There is a good deal of truth in the remark of Schopen-

[1] Barring details, I have held the position here taken, for twenty years. Stumpf, to whom I owe a debt of gratitude for the repeated consideration of my work, has many points of detail (*Tonpsychologie*, Leipsic, 1883) that appeal to me. The view expressed on page 119 of his work, however, is incompatible with the principle of parallelism, my fundamental axiom of research. Compare my note, "Zur Analyse der Tonempfindungen," *Sitzungsberichte der Wiener Akademie*, Vol. 92, II. Abth., p. 1283 (1885).

hauer[1] that music represents the will, and in fact generally in the designation of music as a language of
emotion ; although this is scarcely the whole truth.

2.

Following the precedent of Darwin, H. Berg has
attempted to derive music from the amatory cries of
monkeys.[2] We should be blind not to recognise the
service rendered and enlightenment conveyed by the
work of Darwin and Berg. Even at the present day,
music has power to touch sexual chords, and is, as a
fact, widely made use of in courtship. But as to the
question wherein consists the agreeable quality of
music, Berg makes no satisfactory answer. And seeing that in the matter of harmony he adopts Helmholtz's position of the avoidance of beats and assumes
that the males who howled least disagreeably received
the preference, we may be justified in wondering why
the most intelligent of these animals were not prompted
to maintain silence altogether.

The importance of tracing the connexion of a given
biological phenomenon with the preservation of the
species, and of indicating its phylogenetic origin, cannot be underrated. But we must not imagine that in
having accomplished this we have solved all the problems connected with the phenomenon. Surely no one
will think of explaining the specific sensation of sexual

---

1 Schopenhauer, *Die Welt als Wille und Vorstellung.*
2 H. Berg, *Die Lust an der Musik.* Berlin, 1879.

pleasure by showing its connexion with the preservation
of the species. We should be more likely to acknowledge that the species is preserved because the sensation accompanying sexual indulgence is pleasurable.
Although music may actually *remind* us of the courtship of distant progenitors, it must, if it was ever used
for wooing, have contained at the start some *positive*
agreeable quality, which does not, of course, preclude
its being *re-enforced* at the present time by that memory. To take an analogous case from individual life,
the smell of an oil-lamp which has just been extinguished almost always agreeably reminds me of the
magic lantern which I admired as a child. Yet in itself the smell of the lamp is none the less disgusting
for this reason. Nor does the man who is reminded,
by the scent of roses, of a pleasant experience, believe,
on this account, that the perfume was not previously
agreeable. It has only *gained* by the association.[1]
And if the view referred to cannot sufficiently explain
the agreeable quality of music *per se*, it assuredly can
contribute still less to the solution of special questions, as, for instance, why, in a given case, a fourth
is preferred to a fifth.

3.

A rather partial view of the sensations of tone
would be obtained if we were to consider only the

---

[1] Fechner, notably, has emphasised the significance of association for
æsthetics.

province of speech and music. Sensations of tone are
not only a means of communicating ideas, of express-
ing pleasure and pain, of discriminating between the
voices of men, women, and children ; they are not
alone signals of the exertion or passion experienced
by the person speaking or calling ; they also constitute the means by which we distinguish between large
and small bodies when sounding, between the tread of
large and small animals. The highest tones, the very
ones which the vocal organs of man cannot produce,
presumably are of extreme importance for the determination of the direction from which sounds proceed.[1]
In fact, it is more than likely that these latter functions of sensations of tone antedated, in the animal
world, by a long period, those which merely perform a
part in the social life of animals.

4.

There is no one but will cheerfully acknowledge
the decided advance wrought by Helmholtz in the
analysis of sensations of audition.[2] Following his
principles, we recognise in *noises* combinations of *musical* sounds, of which the number, pitch, and intensity
vary with the time. In *compound* musical sounds, or
clangs, we generally hear, along with the fundamental

[1] Mach, " Bemerkungen über die Function der Ohrmuschel " (*Tröltsch's
Archiv für Ohrenheilkunde*, N. F., Vol. III., p. 72).—Compare also Mach and
Fischer, " Die Reflexion und Brechung des Schalles," *Pogg. Ann.*, Vol. 149,
p. 421.

[2] Helmholtz, *Die Lehre von den Tonempfindungen*, first edition, Bruns-
wick, 1863.

n, the partial tones or harmonics $2n$, $3n$, $4n$, etc., each of which corresponds to simple pendular vibrations. If two such musical sounds, the fundamentals of which correspond to the rates of vibration *n* and *m*, be melodically or harmonically combined, there may result, if certain relations of *n* and *m* are satisfied,[1] a partial coincidence of the harmonics, whereby in the first case the relationship of the two sounds is rendered perceptible, and in the second a diminution of beats is effected. All this cannot be disputed, although it may not be deemed *exhaustive*.

We may also give our assent to Helmholtz's physiological theory of the *auditive organ*. The facts observed on the simultaneous sounding of simple notes make it highly probable that there exist, corresponding to the series of vibration-rates, a series of terminal nervous organs, so that for all the different rates of vibration there are different sympathetic end-organs, each of which responds to only a few, closely adjacent rates of vibration. It is a question of lesser importance whether this function is exercised by the organ of Corti.

5.

If we assume with Helmholtz that all noises admit of being resolved into sensations of tone varying in duration, it is evidently superfluous to seek for a special auditive organ for *noises*. A long time ago (in the

---

[1] The *p*th harmonic of *n* coincides with the *q*th of *m* when $pn = qm$, that is $m = (p/q)\, n$, where *p* and *q* are whole numbers.

winter of 1872–1873) I took up the question of the relation of noises (especially that of sharp reports) to
musical tones, and found that all transitions between
the two may be observed. A tone of one hundred and
twenty-eight full vibrations, heard through a small radial slit in a slowly revolving disc, contracts, when its
duration is reduced to from two to three vibrations, to
a short, sharp concussion (or weak report) of very *indistinct* pitch, while with from four to five vibrations,
the pitch is still perfectly distinct.[1] On the other hand,
with sufficient attention, a pitch, though not a very
definite one, may be detected in a report even when the
latter is produced by an aperiodic motion of the air
(the wave of an electric spark, exploding soap-bubbles
filled with $2\,H+O$). We may easily convince ourselves, furthermore, that in a piano from which the
damper has been lifted, large exploding bubbles mainly
excite to sympathetic vibration the lower strings, while
small ones principally affect the higher strings.   This
fact, it seems clear to me, demonstrates that the same
organ may be the mediator of both tone and noise sensation.   We must imagine that weak aperiodic vibrations of the air having *short* durations excite *all*, though
preferably the *small* and more mobile end-organs, whilst
the powerful and more lasting disturbances of this sort
affect also the larger and heavier end-organs, which
from being less damped perform vibrations of *greater*
amplitude and are thus noticed ; and furthermore that

[1] For full explanation see Appendix II.—*Trans.*

even in the case of comparatively weak *periodic* vibrations of the air, the excitation, by an accumulation of
effects, is manifested in some definite member of the
series of end-organs.[1] The sensation excited by a report of low or high pitch is *qualitatively* the same as
that produced by striking at once a large number of
adjacent piano-keys, only more intense and of shorter
duration. Moreover, in the *single* excitation produced
by a report, the beats connected with periodic inter-
mittent excitations are eliminated.

6.

Yet despite the recognition with which the theory
of Helmholtz has met, there have not been wanting
voices which have called attention to its incomplete-
ness. The lack of a positive factor in the explanation
of harmony has been very generally felt, the mere absence of beats not being regarded as a sufficient and
satisfactory characterisation of harmony. Thus A. v.
Oettingen[2] feels the want of some expressed *positive*
element characteristic of each interval, and refuses to
regard the value of an interval as dependent upon the
physical accident of the overtones contained in the
sounds. He believes that the positive element in question is to be found in the accompanying *remembrance*

[1] I gave an account of part of my experiments, which were a continuation
of Dvorak's researches on the after-images due to variations of excitation
(1870), in the August number of *Lotos*, 1873. (See Appendix II.) I have never
before mentioned the experiments relative to the excitement of piano-tones
by explosions. It will not be amiss, perhaps, if I do so here.—Pfaundler, S.
Exner, Auerbach, Brücke, and others, subsequently treated the same question
in detail.

[2] *Harmoniesystem in dualer Entwicklung* (Dorpat, 1866), p. 30.

of the common fundamental tone (or tonic), as the harmonics of which the composite notes or clangs of the interval have often occurred, or in the accompanying *remembrance* of the common overtone (or phonic)[1] belonging to the two (pp. 40, 47). On the negative side of his criticisms I am in complete agreement with Von Oettingen. But "remembrance" does not quite fill the need of the theory, for consonance and dissonance are not matters of representative activity, but of sensation. My opinion, therefore, is that A. von Oettingen's conception is *physiologically* inadequate. His enunciation of the principle of duality, however, (or of the principle of the tonic and phonic relationship of composite notes), as also his conception of dissonances as indeterminate composite musical sounds admitting of more than one interpretation (p. 224) appear to me to be valuable and positive services to science.[2]

[1] [The lowest of the harmonics common to all I term the coincident or phonic harmonic.—Von Oettingen, *Harmoniesystem in dualer Entwicklung*, p. 32. *Quoted by translator.*]

[2] A popular statement of the principle of duality, of which Euler (*Tentamen novae theoriae musicae*, p. 103), D'Alembert (*Elémens de musique*, Lyons, 1766), and Hauptmann (*Die Natur der Harmonik und Metrik*, Leipsic, 1853, translation by W. E. Heathcote, London, Swan Sonnenschein & Co., 1888), had all a faint inkling, is to be found in my *Popular Scientific Lectures* (Chicago, 1894), under the caption "Symmetry" (originally published in 1872). Perfect symmetry, such as is found in the province of sight, cannot be imagined in music, since sensations of tone do not constitute a symmetrical system.

7.

I myself, as early as 1863[1], and also later,[2] had made some critical remarks on the theory of Helmholtz, and in 1866, in a small work[3] which appeared shortly before that of Von Oettingen, very definitely pointed out some demands which a more perfect theory of the subject would have to satisfy. Since, however, up to the present time my remarks have, to my knowledge, nowhere met with serious consideration, I shall revert to them here at length.

8.

We shall start with the idea that a series of definitely graduated sonant end-organs exists, the members of which, as the rate of vibration increases, successively yield their maximum response, and we shall ascribe to each end-organ its particular (specific) energy. Then there are as many specific energies as there are end-organs, and a like number of rates of vibration auditively distinguishable by us.

Further, we not only *distinguish* between tones, but we assign to them also their *ordinal* places in a series. Of three tones of different pitch, we recognise the middle one immediately as such. We feel immediately which rates of vibration lie near together and

[1] Mach, "Zur Theorie des Gehörorgans" (*Sitzungsberichte der Wiener Akademie*, 1863.

[2] Compare my "Bemerkungen zur Lehre vom räumlichen Sehen" (*Fichte's Zeitschrift für Philosophie*, 1865).

[3] *Einleitung in die Helmholtz'sche Musiktheorie*, Graz, 1866. See the Preface and pp. 23 et seq., 46 and 48.

which lie far apart.   This is readily enough explained
for neighboring tones.   For, if we represent the vibra-
tion-amplitudes of a certain tone symbolically by the
curve *a b c*, Fig. 35, and imagine this curve gradually
moved in the direction of the arrow, then, since necessarily several organs always yield simultaneous re-
sponses, neighboring tones will always have faint,
common excitations.   But *distant* tones also possess a
certain similarity ; and even between the highest and
lowest tones we can detect a resemblance.   Consequently, in accordance with the principle of investigation by which we are guided, we are obliged to assume

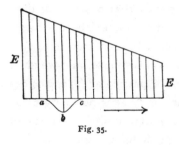

Fig. 35.

in *all* tone-sensations
common factors.   Conse-
quently, again, there cannot be as many specific
energies as there are distinguishable tones.   For
the understanding of the
facts with which we are

here concerned, it *suffices* to assume only two energies,
which are excited in different proportions by different
rates of vibration.   Further complexity of the sensations of tone is not excluded by these facts, but on the
contrary is rendered probable by phenomena to be discussed later.

Careful *psychological* analysis of the tonal series
leads immediately to this view.   But even supposing
we assume a special energy for every rod of Corti, and

reflect that these energies are similar to one another, that is, contain common elements, virtually we arrive at the same conception. For let us assume, merely in order to have a definite picture before us, that, in the transition from the lowest to the highest rates of vibration, the tonal sensation varies similarly to the color-sensation in passing from pure red to pure yellow, say by the gradual admixture of yellow. We can fully retain, on this view, the idea that there is for every distinguishable rate of vibration a special appropriate end-organ; but in that case not absolutely different energies, but always the same two energies, only in different proportions, are disengaged by the different organs.[1]

9.

How does it happen, now, that a number of notes simultaneously sounded are *distinguished*, seeing that we should naturally expect them to blend into a single sensation; or that two tones of different pitch do not blend to a *mixed tone* of intermediate pitch? The fact that this does not happen, lends a still more definite shape to the conception which we have to form. The case is probably similar to that of a graduated series of mixed reds and yellows situated at different points of space, which are likewise distinguished

---

[1] The view that different end-organs respond to different rates of vibration is too well supported by the production of beats by neighboring tones, and by other facts adduced by Helmholtz, and, upon the whole, too valuable for the comprehension of the phenomena, to be again relinquished. The view here presented utilises the facts disclosed, notably by Hering, in the analysis of color-sensations.

and do not blend. As a fact, the sensation which ensues when the attention passes from one tone to another is similar to that which accompanies the wandering of the fixation-point in the field of vision. The tonal series is an analogue of space, but of a space of *one* dimension limited in both directions and exhibiting no symmetry like that, for instance, of a straight line running from right to left in a direction perpendicular to the median plane. It more resembles a vertical right line, or one running from the front to the rear in the median plane. But while colors are not confined to certain points in space, but may move about, which is the reason we so easily separate space-sensations from color-sensations, the case is different with tone-sensations. A particular tone-sensation can occur only at a particular point of the said one-dimensional space, on which the attention must in each case be fixed if the tone-sensation in question is to be distinctly perceived. We may now imagine that different tone-sensations have their origin in different parts of the auditive substance, or that, in addition to the two energies whose ratio determines the timbre of high and deep tones, a third exists, which is similar to the sensation of innervation, and which comes into play in the fixation of tones. Or both conditions might occur together. At present it may be regarded as neither possible nor necessary to come to a conclusion in the matter.

That the province of tone-sensation offers an analogy to space, and to a space having no symmetry, unconsciously expresses itself in language. We speak of high tones and deep tones, not of right tones and left tones, although our musical instruments suggest the latter designation as a very natural one.

In one of my earliest publications[1] I supported the view that the fixation of tones was connected with a varying tension of the *tensor tympani.* I am now unable to maintain this view in the light of subsequent observations and experiments which I have made. Nevertheless, the space-analogy does not fall to the ground for this reason; but merely the appropriate *physiological* element remains to be discovered.[2]

[1] *Zur Theorie des Gehörorgans,* 1863.

[2] The supposition that the processes in the larynx during singing have had something to do with the formation of the tonal series I likewise noticed in my work of 1863, but did not find it tenable. Singing is connected in too extrinsic and accidental a manner with hearing to bear out such an hypothesis. I can hear and imagine tones far beyond the range of my own voice. In listening to an orchestral performance with all the parts, or in having an hallucination of such a performance, it is impossible for me to think that my understanding of this broad and complicated sound-fabric has been effected by my *one* larynx, which is, moreover, no very practised singer. I consider the sensations which, in listening to singing, are doubtless occasionally noticed in the larynx, a matter of subsidiary importance, like the pictures of the keys touched which, when I was more in practice, sprang up immediately into my imagination on hearing a performance on the piano or organ. When I imagine music, I always distinctly hear the notes. Music can no more come into being merely through the motor sensations accompanying musical performances than a deaf man can hear by watching the movements of players. I cannot, therefore, agree with Stricker on this point. (Comp. Stricker: *Du langage et de la musique.* Paris, 1885).

Different is my opinion with regard to Stricker's views on language. (Comp. Stricker, *Die Sprachvorstellungen,* Vienna, 1880.) It is true that in my own case words of which I think reverberate loudly in my ear. Moreover, I have no doubt that thoughts may be directly excited by the ringing of a housebell, by the whistle of a locomotive, etc., and that small children and even dogs understand words which they cannot repeat. Nevertheless, I have been convinced by Stricker that the ordinary and most familiar, though not the only possible way by which speech is comprehended, is really *motor,* and

10.

The analogy between fixing the eyes on points in space and fixing the attention on tones, I have repeatedly illustrated by experiments, which I shall cite again here. One and the same combination of two tones sounds different according as we fix our attention upon the one or the other. Combinations 1 and 2 in the annexed cut have a perceptibly different char-

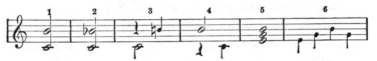

acter according as we fix our attention on the higher or on the lower note. Persons not able to transfer their attention arbitrarily will be helped by having

that we should be badly off if we were without it. I can cite corroborations of this view from my own experience. I frequently see strangers who are endeavoring to follow my remarks, slightly moving their lips. If a person tells me his place of residence and I omit to repeat the street and number of the house after him, I am certain to forget the address, but with the exercise of this precautionary measure, I retain it perfectly in memory. A friend told me recently that he had stopped reading the Indian drama *Urvasi*, because he had great difficulty in spelling out the names, and consequently could not retain them in memory. The dream of the deaf-mute, which Stricker relates, is intelligible only from his point of view. In fact, on calm reflexion this seemingly paradoxical relation is by no means so remarkable. The extent to which our thoughts move in accustomed and routine channels is shown by the surprise produced by witticisms. Good jokes would be more frequent if our minds moved less in *ruts.* To many the obvious collatéral meanings of words never suggest themselves. Who, for example, in using the names Smith, Baker, or Taylor thinks of the occupations designated! To adduce an analogous example from a different field, I may state (comp. p. 51) that I immediately recognise writing reflected in a mirror and *accompanying* its original, as symmetrically congruent with the latter, although I am not able to read it directly, because of my having learned writing by *motor* methods, with my *right* hand. I can also best illustrate by this example why I do not agree with Stricker in regard to music: music is related to speech as ornament is to writing.

one note sound later than the other. This then draws the attention after it. With a little practice it is possible to decompose a chord (as, for instance, 5) into its elements and to hear the constituent tones by themselves (as in 6). These and the following experiments are better and more convincingly carried out upon a physharmonica than on a piano, owing to the greater duration of the tones.

Especially astonishing is the phenomenon produced when we cause one note of a cord, on which the attention is fixed, to be damped. The attention then passes over to the note nearest to it, which comes out with the distinctness of a note that has just been struck. The impression made by the experiment is quite similar to that which we receive when, absorbed in work, we suddenly hear the regular striking of the clock emerge into distinctness after having entirely vanished from consciousness. In the latter case the entire tonal effect passes the threshold of consciousness, whilst in the former a part is augmented. If in 7, for example, we fix the attention upon the upper

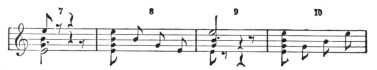

note, letting go, successively from above, the keys damping the other notes, the effect obtained is approximately that of 8. If, in 9, we fix the attention on the lowest note, and proceed in the reverse order, we obtain the impression represented in 10. The same chordal combination sounds quite different according to the part on which the attention is fixed. If, in 11 or 12, I fix my attention on the upper note,

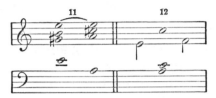

the *timbre* alone appears to be altered. But if in 11, the attention be fixed upon the bass, the entire acoustic mass will seem to sink in depth; while in 12 it will appear to rise if we regard closely the succession e–f. It is quite evident, in fine, that *chords* act the part of *clangs* (or compound notes embracing both fundamentals and harmonics). The facts here advanced remind us strongly of the changing impression received when, in observing an ornamental design, the attention is alternately fixed on different points.

We may also recall to mind here the involuntary wandering of the attention which takes place during the continuous and uniform sounding of a note on the harmonium, where if the note lasts several minutes, all the overtones will of themselves successively emerge into full distinctness.[1] The process appears to point to a sort of fatigue for the note on which the attention has long been fixed. This fatigue, moreover, is ren-

---

[1] Compare my *Einleitung in die Helmholtz'sche Musiktheorie*, p. 29

dered quite probable by an experiment which I have
described at length in another place.[1]

The relations we have here been describing, touching sensations of tone, might be illustrated perhaps
more palpably by some such parallel as the following.
Suppose that our two eyes were capable of only a single
movement, that they could only follow, by changing
motions of symmetrical convergence, the
points of a horizontal straight line lying
in the median plane ; and suppose that
the nearest points on this line fixed by
the eyes were pure red, and those farthest
away, corresponding to the position of
parallelism, were pure yellow, while between them lay all intermediate shades ;
then the system of sight-sensations so

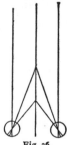

Fig. 36.

constructed would quite palpably resemble the facts
presented by sensations of tone.

II.

On the view hitherto developed, an important fact,
which we shall now state, remains unintelligible,
though its explanation is absolutely necessary if the
theory is to lay any claim to completeness. If two
series of tones be begun at two different points on the
scale, but be made to maintain throughout the same
ratios of vibration, we shall recognise in both the same

[1] Compare my *Grundlinien der Lehre von den Bewegungsempfindungen*,
p. 58.

melody, by a mere act of sensation, just as readily and immediately as we recognise in two geometrically similar figures, similarly situated, the same form. Like melodies, differently situated on the scale, might be denominated tonal constructs of *like tonal form*, or they might be denominated *similar* tonal constructs, from their space-analogues.

Even in a series of only two tones, the sameness of the vibrational ratios is at once recognised. Thus the series c–f, d–g, e–a, etc., which have all the same vibrational *ratios* (3:4), are immediately recognised as *like intervals*, as *fourths*. Such is the fact, in its simplest form. The ability to pick out and recognise intervals is the first thing required of the student of music who is desirous of becoming thoroughly familiar with his province.

In a little work,[1] well worth reading, by Mr. E. Kulke, mention is made, bearing on this point, of an original method of instruction by P. Cornelius—a description of which I will here complete from Kulke's own lips. According to Cornelius, it is a wonderful help in the recognition of intervals to make note of particular pieces of music, folk-songs, etc., which *begin* with these intervals. The Overture to Tannhäuser, for example, begins with a fourth. If I hear a fourth I at once remark that the series of tones is the same as that beginning the Overture to Tannhäuser and

---

[1] E. Kulke, *Ueber die Umbildung der Melodie. Ein Beitrag zur Entwicklungslehre.* Prague. Calve. 1884.

by this means recognise the interval. In like manner, the Overture to Fidelio may be used as the representative of the third ; and so on. This excellent device, which I have put to the test in my lectures on acoustics and have found very effective, apparently complicates matters. One would naturally suppose that it would be easier to make note of an interval than of a melody. Nevertheless, a melody offers a greater hold to memory than does an interval, just as an individual countenance is more easily remarked and associated with a name than is a certain facial angle or a nose. Every one makes note of faces and associates with them names ; but Leonardo da Vinci arranged noses in a system.

And as every interval in a *series* of tones is made perceptible in characteristic manner, so it is with the *harmonic* combinations of tones. Every third, every fourth, every major or minor triad has its characteristic color, by which it is recognised independently of the pitch of the fundamental, and independently of the number of beats, which rapidly increase with increasing pitch.

A tuning-fork held before *one* ear is very feebly heard by the *other* ear. If two slightly discordant, beating tuning-forks are held in front of the same ear, the beats are very distinct. But if one of the forks be placed before one ear, and the other before the other, the beats will be greatly *weakened*. Two forks of harmonic interval always sound slightly *rougher* before

one ear.   But the character of the harmony is preserved when one is placed before each ear.[1]   Discord
also remains quite perceptible in this experiment.
Harmony and discord are certainly not determined by
beats *alone.*

In melodic as well as in harmonic combinations,
notes whose rates of vibrations bear to one another
some simple ratio, are distinguished (1) by their *agree-
ableness,* and (2), by a sensation *characteristic* of this
ratio.   As for the agreeable quality, there is no deny-
ing but this is *partly* explained by the coincidence of
the overtones, and, in the case of harmonic combination, by the consequent effacement of the beats, re-
sulting always where the ratios of the numbers representing the vibrations satisfy certain simple conditions.
But the experienced and unprejudiced student of music is not entirely satisfied with this explanation.   He
is disturbed by the preponderant rôle accorded to the
accident of acoustic color, and notices that tones further stand to each other in a positive relation of *contrast,* like colors, except that, in the case of colors, no
such definite agreeable relations can be specified.

The fact that a sort of contrast really does exist
among tones is almost forced upon our notice.   A
smooth, unchanging tone is something very unpleas-
ing and characterless, like a single uniform color enveloping our entire surroundings.   A lively effect is

---

[1] Compare Fechner, *Ueber einige Verhältnisse des binocularen Sehens,*
Leipsic, 1860, p. 536.

produced only on the addition of a second tone, a second color. In like manner, if we cause a tone gradually to mount in pitch, as in experiments with the siren, all contrast is lost. Contrast exists, however, between tones farther apart, and not merely between those immediately following one another, as the accompanying example will show. Passage 2 sounds

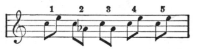

quite different after 1 from what it does alone, 3 sounds different from 2, and even 5 different from 4 immediately following 3.

12.

Let us turn now to the second point, the *characteristic sensation* corresponding to each interval, and ask if this can be explained on the current theory. If a fundamental n be melodically or harmonically combined with its third m, the fifth harmonic of the *first* note ($5n$) will coincide with the *fourth* of the second note ($4m$). This, according to the theory of Helmholtz, is the *common feature* characterising all third-combinations. If I combine the notes C and E, or F and A, representing their harmonics in the cut on the next page, then, as a fact, in the one case the harmonics marked $\lfloor$ and in the other those marked $\dagger$ coincide; and in both cases the coincidence is between the fifth harmonic of the lower and the fourth harmonic of the higher note. Be it noted, however, that this common feature exists solely for the *understanding*, being the result of a purely physical and intellectual analysis, and has nothing to do with *sensation.* For sensation the real coincidence in the first case is between the ē's, and in the second between the ā's, which are entirely different notes. On the assumption that there

C	c	g	c̄	e	ḡ	b-flat	c̄̄
n	*2n*	*3n*	*4n*	*5n*	*6n*	*7n*	*8n*

E	e	b	e̱	g-sharp	b̄	d̄̄	ē̱
m	*2m*	*3m*	*4m*	*5m*	*6m*	*7m*	*8m*

F	f	c̄	f̄	a	c̄̄	e-flat	f̄̄
n	*2n*	*3n*	*4n*	*5n*	*6n*	*7n*	*8n*

A	a	e	a	c-sharp	ē̱	ḡ̱	a
m	*2m*	*3m*	*4m*	*5m*	*6m*	*7m*	*8m*

exists for every distinguishable rate of vibration an appurtenant specific energy, we are obliged, more than on any other theory, to ask where is the common component of sensation hidden that characterises every third combination?

I must insist on this distinction of mine not being regarded as a piece of pedantic hair-splitting. I propounded the question involving it about twenty years ago, at the same time with my question as to wherein physiological similarity of form, as distinguished from geometrical, consisted ; and it is not a whit more un- necessary than was that, whose superfluity, too, in the issue, was disproved. If we are to suffer a *physical* or *mathematical* characteristic of the third interval to stand as a mark of the third-*sensation*, then we should content ourselves, as Euler did,[1] with the coincidence of every fourth and fifth vibration—a conception which was, after all, not so bad, provided it could be supposed that sound continued its course in the nerve-tracts, also, as *periodic* motion, a view which even A. Seebeck (*Pogg. Ann.*, Vol. 68) regarded as possible. With re- gard to this particular point, Helmholtz's coincidence of $5n$ and $4m$ is in no respect less symbolical and does not offer greater enlightenment.

13.

So far I have presented my arguments with the conviction that I should not find it necessary to make a single retrograde step of importance. This feeling does not accompany me in the same measure in the development of the following hypothesis, which, in all its essential features, was suggested to me a long time ago. Yet the hypothesis may at least serve to clear up and illustrate, from the positive side also, the requirement which I believe a more complete theory of tone-sensations is bound to meet.

We will begin by supposing that it is an extremely

---

[1] Euler, *Tentamen novae theoriae musicae*, Petropoli, 1789, p. 36.

important vital condition for an animal of simple organisation to perceive slight periodic motions of the medium in which it lives. If (owing to the relatively excessive size of its organs, and its consequent lack of receptivity for such rapid changes) its attention is too sluggishly transferred, the period of the impinging vibrations is too short, or their amplitude too small, to permit the *single* phases of the excitation to enter consciousness, it may nevertheless be possible under certain conditions for the animal to perceive the *accumulated* sensation-effects of the oscillatory excitation. The organ of hearing will outstrip the organ of touch.[1] Now an end-organ capable of vibration (say an auditory cilium) responds, by virtue of its physical qualities, not to *every* rate of vibration, nor to *one* only, but ordinarily to *several*, at a considerable distance apart.[2] Therefore, as soon as the whole continuum of vibrational rates between certain limits becomes of importance for the animal, a small number of end-organs no longer suffice, but the need of a whole series of such organs of graduated sonancy arises. The organ of Corti is regarded as such a system.

It can hardly be expected, however, that a member of Corti's organ will respond to only *one* rate of

[1] It is questionable therefore whether animals which have so small a measure of time that their voluntary movements produce a musical note hear in the ordinary sense, or whether with them that is not rather touch which makes on us the impression of hearing. Compare, for example, the admirable experiments and observations of V. Graber (" Die Chordotonalen Organe," *Arch. für Microskop. Anat.*, XX., p. 506).—Compare also my *Bewegungsempfindungen*, p. 123.

[2] As V. Hensen, for example, has observed.

vibration. On the contrary, we must suppose that it responds with enfeebled but graduated intensity (perhaps from being divided by nodes) to the rates of vibration $2n$, $3n$, $4n$, etc., as also to the rates of vibration $n/2$, $n/3$, $n/4$, etc. Inasmuch as the assumption of a special energy for each rate of vibration has proved untenable, we may imagine, agreeably to remarks made above, that in the first place, only two sensation-energies, Dull (D) and Clear (C), are excited. The resultant sensation we will represent *symbolically* (somewhat as we do in mixed colors) by $pD + qC$; or, making $p + q = 1$ and regarding q as a function $f(n)$ of the rate of vibration,[1] by $[1 - f(n)]$ $D + f(n) C$. The sensation arising will now correspond to the *number of the vibrations* producing the oscillatory excitation, on whatever member of Corti's series the excitation may light. And consequently the current conception will not be materially disturbed by the new hypothesis. For, since the member R_n responds most powerfully to n, and only in a much more enfeebled degree to $2n$, $3n$, or to $n/2$, $n/3$, R_n vibrating with n even in case of an aperiodic impulse, therefore the sensation $[1 - f(n)] D + f(n) C$ will still be *predominantly* associated with R_n.

Well-attested cases of double hearing (compare Stumpf, *loc. cit.*, p. 206, et seq.) point forcibly to the conclusion that the ratios in which the energies D and C are disengaged are dependent upon the *end-organ*,

[1] Thus, to take a very simple example, we might make $f(n) = k \cdot \log n$.

and not upon the rate of vibration—a conclusion which would also not affect our conception.

A member R_n, accordingly, responds powerfully to n, and also, though more weakly, to $2n$, $3n$, ... , $n/2$, $n/3$ . . . . with the sensations belonging to these rates of vibration.   It is, however, extremely improbable that *exactly* the same sensation is excited whether R_n responds to n, or whether $R_{\frac{n}{2}}$ responds to n.   On the contrary, it is probable that every time the members of Corti's series respond to a *partial tone*, the sensation receives a weak *supplementary coloring*, which we will represent symbolically, for the fundamental tone by Z_1, for the overtones by Z_2, Z_3, ..., and for the undertones by $Z_{\frac{1}{2}}$, $Z_{\frac{1}{3}}$, ...   On this supposition, sensations of tone would be somewhat *richer* in composition than would follow from the formula $[1 - f(n)] D + f(n) C$.   The sensations which Corti's series, as excited by the fundamentals, yields, constitute a province with the supplementary coloring Z_1, the excitation of the same series by the first overtone yields a special province of sensation with the supplementary coloring Z_2, etc.   The Z's may be either unchanging elements, or may themselves, again, consist of two components, U and V, and form series representable by $[1 - f(n)] U + f(n) V$.   But at present the decision on this last point is immaterial.

It is true that the *physiological* elements Z_1, Z_2, ... have yet to be found.   Yet the very perception that they have to be *sought* seems to me of importance.

Let us see what form the province of tone-sensations would take on if we regarded $Z_1, Z_2, \ldots$ as given.

Our example is a melodic or harmonic major-third combination, whose rates of vibration are $n = 4p$ and $m = 5p$; the lowest of the overtones common to the two is $5n = 4m = 20p$, the highest of the undertones common to the two is p. Then we obtain the following table :[1]

The members of the Corti series:	R_p	R_{4p}	R_{5p}	R_{20p}
When the notes $4p$ and $5p$ do not contain overtones — respond to the rates of vibration:	$4p, 5p$	$4p$	$5p$	$4p = \dfrac{20p}{5}$ $5p = \dfrac{20p}{4}$
with the supplementary sensations:	Z_4, Z_5	Z_1	Z_1	$Z_{\frac{1}{5}}, Z_{\frac{1}{4}}$
When the notes $4p$ and $5p$ contain overtones — they also respond to the rates of vibration:		$20p = 5\,(4p)$	$20p = 4\,(5p)$	
with the supplementary sensations:		Z_5	Z_4	

Thus in the third combination, the supplementary sensations Z_4, Z_5, and $Z_{\frac{1}{4}}$, $Z_{\frac{1}{5}}$, which are characteristic of the third, make their appearance even when the

---

[1] It will be observed that the analysis of the tone-sensations here offered follows the same path as the current analysis of color-sensations. In both cases, inquirers started with the view that to the endless physical differences presented in the world there corresponded endless physiological differences. Conformably to the principle of parallelism, the number of the sensation-elements has in both cases been reduced.

notes contain no overtones, while the former (Z_4, Z_5) are strengthened when, either in the open air or at least in the ear, overtones do occur. The diagram may be easily generalised to include any interval.

These supplementary colorings, though scarcely noticeable in single tones, or in running continuously through the scale, become conspicuous in combinations of tones having certain rates of vibrations, just as the contrasts of faintly colored, almost white lights become vivid when these are brought together. And, furthermore, the same contrast-colorings always correspond to the same ratios of vibrations, no matter what the pitch.

In this manner it is intelligible how tones may receive, by melodic and harmonic combination with *others*, the most varied colorings, which are wanting to them when *singly* sounded.

The elements Z_1, Z_2 . . . must not be conceived as unvarying and fixed in number. On the contrary, it is to be supposed that the number of perceptible Z's depends on the organisation, on the training of the ear, and on the attention. According to this conception, the ear does not directly cognise ratios of vibrations but only the supplementary colorings conditioned by these. The tonal series symbolically represented by $[1 - f(n)]D + f(n)C$ is not infinite but limited. Since $f(n)$ may vary between the values 0 and 1, D and C are the extremes, the terminal sensations corresponding to the lowest and highest tones. If the number of vibrations sinks considerably below or rises considerably above that of the fundamental of the longest and the shortest Corti fibre, a weak response only will take place, but no alteration of the quality of the sensation. Likewise, the sensation due to the *interval* must disappear in the neighborhood of the limits of hearing; first, because in general differences between sensations of tone cease at this point, and, further, because at the upper boundary the members of the Corti series susceptible of being excited by the undertones, are lacking, as are also at the lower boundary those which react on the overtones.

14.

Passing in review again the conception gained, we see that with few exceptions the conclusions reached by Helmholtz may be all retained. Noises and composite sounds may be decomposed into musical tones. For every perceptible rate of vibration there corresponds a particular nervous end-organ. In place of the numerous specific energies required by this theory, however, we substitute but *two*, which render the relationship of all tonal sensations intelligible, and by the rôle which we assign to the attention, likewise enable us to keep perceptually *distinct*, several tones when sounded together. By the hypothesis of the multiple response of the members of the Corti series, and that of supplementary acoustic colorings, the sig-

nificance of accidental acoustic tints is diminished,
and we get a glimpse of the direction in which, notably on the ground of musical facts, the *positive* characteristics of intervals are to be sought.   Finally, by
the latter conception, Von Oettingen's principle of
duality acquires a basis, which might perhaps com-
mend itself to this investigator himself better than his
assumption of "memory"; while at the same time it
becomes manifest why the duality cannot be a perfect
symmetry.

15.

To a person accustomed to looking at things from
the point of view of the theory of evolution, the high
development of modern music as well as the spontaneous and sudden appearance of great musical talent
seem, at first glance, a most singular and problematic
phenomenon.   What could this remarkable development of the power of hearing have had to do with the
preservation of the species?   Does it not far exceed
the measure of the necessary or the useful?   What can
possibly be the significance of a fine discriminative
sense of pitch?   Of what use to us is a perceptive
sense of intervals, or of the acoustic colorings of orchestral music?

As a matter of fact, the same question may be proposed with reference to every art, no matter from what
province of sense its material is derived.   The question is pertinent, also, with regard to the intelligence

of a Newton, an Euler, or their like, which apparently far transcends the necessary measure. But the question is most obvious with reference to music, which satisfies no practical need and for the most part depicts nothing. Music, however, is closely allied to the decorative arts. In order to be able to see, a person must have the power of distinguishing the *directions* of lines. Having a *fine* power of distinction, such a person may acquire, as a sort of collateral product of his education, a feeling for *agreeable* combinations of lines. The case is the same with the sense of *color-harmony* following upon the development of the power of distinguishing colors, and so, too, it undoubtedly is with respect to music.

We must bear in mind that talent and genius, however gigantic their achievements may appear to us, constitute but a slight departure from normal endowment. Talent may be resolved into the possession of psychical power slightly above the average in a certain province. And as for genius, it is talent supplemented by a capacity of adaptation extending beyond the youthful period, and by the retention of freedom to overstep routine barriers. The naïveté of the child delights us, and produces almost always the impression of genius. But this impression as a rule quickly disappears, and we perceive that the very same utterances which, as adults, we are wont to ascribe to freedom, have their source, in the child, in a lack of fixed character.

Talent and genius, as Weismann has aptly shown,[1] do not make their appearance slowly and by degrees in the course of generations ; nor can they be the result of accumulated effort and practice on the part of ancestors ; but they manifest themselves spontaneously and suddenly. Taken in connexion with the preceding, this, too, is intelligible, if we will but reflect that descendants are not exact reproductions of their ancestors, but exhibit the qualities of the latter with some variations, now slightly diminished, now slightly augmented in amount.

[1] Weismann, *Ueber die Vererbung*, Jena, 1883, (English translation, Clarendon Press, Oxford, 1889,) p. 43.

PHYSICS.

INFLUENCE OF THE PRECEDING INVESTIGATIONS ON THE MODE OF ITS CONCEPTION.[1]

I.

WHAT gain does physics derive from the preceding investigations? In the first place, a very wide-spread *prejudice* is removed, and with it, a *barrier*. There is no rift between the psychical and the physical, no *within* and *without*, no *sensation* to which an outward, different *thing* corresponds. There is but *one kind of elements*, out of which this supposititious within and without is formed—elements which are themselves within and without according to the light in which, for the time being, they are viewed.

2.

The world of *sense* belongs to the physical and the psychical domain *alike*. As, in studying the be-

1 I have partly discussed the questions considered in this chapter, before. (See my *Erhaltung der Arbeit*, Prague, Calve, 1872, and also the essay on "The Economical Nature of Physical Inquiry," first published in 1882, and now in my *Popular Scientific Lectures*, Chicago, 1894.) With regard to the idea of concepts as labor-saving instruments, Prof. W. James, of Harvard University, has, in conversation, directed my attention to points of agreement between my writings and his essay on "The Sentiment of Rationality" (*Mind*, Vol. IV., p. 317, July, 1879). This essay, written with refreshing vigor and impartiality, will be perused by every one with pleasure and profit.

havior of gases, by disregarding variations of temperature we reach Mariotte's law, but by expressly considering them, Gay Lussac's, while throughout our
object of investigation remains *the same*, so, too, we
study *physics* in its broadest signification when in
searching into the connexions of the world of sense
we *leave the body entirely out of account*, whereas we
pursue the *psychology of the senses* when we direct our
main attention to the body and above all to *our* nervous system. *Our* body, like every other, is part of
the world of sense ; the boundary-line between the
physical and the psychical is solely practical and conventional. If, for the higher purposes of science, we
erase this dividing-line, and consider all connexions
as *equivalent*, new paths of investigation cannot fail to
be opened up.

3.

We must regard it as an additional gain that the
physicist is now no longer overawed by the traditional
intellectual implements of physics. If ordinary "matter" must be regarded merely as a highly natural,
unconsciously constructed mental symbol for a complex of sensuous elements, much more must this be
the case with the artificial hypothetical atoms and
molecules of physics and chemistry. The value of
these implements for their special, limited purposes
is not one whit destroyed. As before, they remain
still economical symbolisations of the world of experience. But we have as little right to expect from them,

as from the symbols of algebra (to use an apposite analogue), more than we have put into them, and certainly not more enlightenment and revelation than from experience itself. We are on our guard now, even in the province of physics, against overestimating the value of our symbols. Still less, therefore, should the monstrous idea ever enter our heads of employing atoms to explain psychical processes; seeing that atoms are but the symbols of certain peculiar complexes of sensuous elements which we meet with in the narrow domain of *physics.*

4.

The sciences may be distinguished according to the matter of which they treat, as also by their manner of treating it. Further, all science has for its aim *the representation of facts in thought,* either for *practical* ends, or for removing *intellectual* discomfort. Resuming the terminology of the "Introductory Remarks," science, it may be said, arises where in any manner the elements ABC . . . or the elements KLM . . . are reproduced or representatively mimicked by the elements $\alpha\beta\gamma$ . . . , or the latter by one another. For example, physics (in its broadest signification) arises through representatively reproducing by $\alpha\beta\gamma$ . . . the elements ABC in their relations to one another; the physiology or psychology of the *senses,* through reproducing in like manner the relations of ABC . . . to KLM . . . ; physiology, through reproducing the relations of KLM . . . to one another and to ABC . . . ; while the reproducing of the $\alpha\beta\gamma$ . . . themselves by other $\alpha\beta\gamma$ leads to the psychological sciences proper.

Now one might be of the opinion, say, with respect to physics, that the portrayal of the sense-given *facts* is of less importance than the atoms, forces, and laws by which they are portrayed, and which form, so to speak, the *nucleus* of the sense-given facts. But un-biassed reflexion discloses that every *practical* and *intellectual* need is satisfied the moment our thoughts have acquired the power to represent the facts of the senses completely. Such representation, consequently, is the *end and aim* of physics; while atoms, forces, and laws are merely *means* facilitating the representation. Their value extends as far, and as far only, as the help they afford.

5.

Our knowledge of a natural phenomenon, say of an earthquake, is as complete as possible when our thoughts so marshal before the eye of the mind all the relevant sense-given facts of the case that they may be regarded almost as a *substitute* for the latter, and the facts appear to us as old familiar figures, having no power to occasion surprise. When, in imagination, we hear the subterranean thunders, feel the oscillation of the earth, figure to ourselves the sensation produced by the rising and sinking of the ground, the cracking of the walls, the falling of the plaster, the

movement of the furniture and the pictures, the stop-
ping of the clocks, the rattling and smashing of win-
dows, the wrenching of the door-posts, the jamming
of the doors ; when we see in mind the oncoming un-
dulation passing over a forest as lightly as a gust of
wind over a field of grain, breaking the branches of
the trees ; when we see the town enveloped in a cloud
of dust, hear the bells begin to ring in the towers ;
further, when the subterranean processes, which are
at present unknown to us, shall stand out in full sensuous reality before our eyes, so that we shall see the
earthquake advancing as we see a waggon approaching
in the distance till finally we feel the earth shaking beneath our feet,—then more insight than this we cannot
have, and more we do not require. If we cannot combine the partial facts in their right and required proportions without the aid of certain auxiliary conceptions drawn from mathematics, it yet remains true that
the latter merely enable our thoughts to grasp gradually and piecemeal what they are unable to grasp all
at once. These auxiliary conceptions would be de-
void of value, could we not reach, by their help, the
graphic representation of the sense-given facts.

When I see in thought a white beam of light which
falls upon a prism issue forth in a fan-shaped band of
colors having certain angles which I can specify beforehand ; when I see its real spectrum-image, obtained upon a screen by interposing a lens, and in that
image, at points determinable in advance, Fraunhofer's

lines; when I see, in my mind, how these self-same
lines alter their position on the prism being turned,
on its substance being changed, or on the thermom-
eter in contact with it altering its register, then I know
all that I can require. All auxiliary conceptions, laws,
and formulæ, are but quantitative norms, regulating
my sensory representation of the facts. The latter is
the *end*, the former are the *means*.

6.

The adaptation of thoughts to facts, accordingly,
is the aim of all scientific research. In this, science
only deliberately and consciously pursues what in daily
life goes on unnoticed and of its own accord. As soon
as we become capable of self-observation, we find our
thoughts, in large measure, already adjusted to the
facts. Our thoughts marshal the elements before us
in groups copying the order of the sense-given facts.
But the limited supply of the mental elements cannot
keep pace with the constantly augmenting sweep of
experience. Almost every new fact necessitates a new
adaptation, which finds its expression in the operation
known as *judgment*.

This process of judgment is easily followed in children. A child, on its first visit from the town to the
country, strays, for instance, into a large meadow,
looks about, and says wonderingly: "We are in a
ball. The world is a blue ball."[1] Here we have two

---

[1] This case is not fictitious, but was observed in my three-year old child.

judgments. What is the process accompanying their formation? In the first instance, the existing percept or sense-given image of the company "we" is broadened into a new representative image by union with the similarly existing percept of a ball. Likewise, in the second judgment, the image of the "world" (i.e., all the objects of the environment) is supplemented by combination with the image of an enveloping blue ball (the percept of which must also have been present, since otherwise the name for it would have been wanting). A judgment is thus always a supplementing or amendment of the deficiencies of a sensuous percept to represent completely a sensuous fact. If the judgment can be expressed in *words*, then the new percept is never more than a combination of formerly established memory-images, which can also be elicited in other persons by words.

The process of judgment, therefore, in the present case consists in the enrichment, extension, and supplementation of existing sensuous percepts by *other* existing sensuous percepts, agreeably to the requirements of definite sense-given facts. If the process is over with, and the image has assumed a familiar shape, making its appearance in consciousness as a distinct and intact product, then we have no longer to do with a judgment but merely with a phenomenon of *memory*. To the forming of such "intuitive knowledge," as Locke calls it, natural science and mathematics mainly owe their growth. Consider, for example, the follow-

ing statements: (1) the tree has a root; (2) the frog
has no claws; (3) the caterpillar is transformed into a
butterfly; (4) weak sulphuric acid dissolves zinc; (5)
friction electrifies glass; (6) an electric current de-
flects a magnetic needle; (7) a cube has six surfaces,
eight corners, twelve edges. The first statement em-
bodies a spatial extension of the percept tree, the
second a correction of a percept too hastily generalised
from habit, the third, fourth, fifth, and sixth embody
temporal extensions of their respective representations. The seventh proposition is an example of geometrical "intuition."

7.

Intuitive knowledge of the sort just described, impresses itself upon the memory and makes its appearance there in the form of recollections which spontaneously supplement every fact presented by the
senses. But the facts not being all alike, only their
common elements are emphasised, and so we reach a
principle which holds a paramount place in memory—
the principle of *broadest possible generalisation* or *continuity*. On the other hand, if memory is to satisfy
the requirements made by the dissimilarities of facts,
and be of real practical use, it must conform to the
principle of *sufficient differentiation*. Even the animal
is reminded, by soft, bright red and yellow fruits (seen
without exertion on the tree), of their *sweet* taste, and
by green hard fruits (which are seen with difficulty), of

their *sour* taste. The insect-hunting monkey snatches at everything that buzzes and flies, but avoids the yellow and black fly, the wasp. Here we have expressed, distinctly enough, the combined effort for greatest possible *generalisation and continuity* and for *practically sufficient differentiation* of memory. And both ends are attained by the same means, *the selection and emphasis of those particular elements of the sensuous perception* which are determinative of the direction which the thought must pursue to suit the experience. The physicist proceeds in quite an analogous manner, when he says (generalising) : All transparent solids refract incident light towards the perpendicular, and when he adds (differentiating) : amorphous bodies and isomeric crystals simply, the rest doubly.

8.

A considerable portion of mental adaptation takes place unconsciously and involuntarily, under the natural guidance of the facts presented to the senses. If this adaptation has become sufficiently comprehensive to embrace the vast majority of the occurring facts, and subsequently we come upon a fact which runs violently counter to the customary course of our thought without our being able to discover at once the determinative factor likely to lead to a *new* differentiation, then a *problem* arises. The new, unusual, and marvellous acts as a stimulus, which irresistibly attracts the attention. Practical considerations, or even bare intellectual discomfort, may engender a volitional frame of mind requiring the removal of the contradiction, or a consequent new mental adaptation.   Thus arises *purposive* thought-adaptation, *investigation.*

For example, we have all, at some time or another, quite contrary to the common run of our experience, observed a lever or pulley lifting by means of a small weight a large weight.   We seek the differentiating factor, which in the sensuous phenomenon itself is not immediately given.   We compare a number of different instances falling under the same category, note the varying influences exerted by the *weights* and the *arms of the lever*, and *then*, only after having mastered by strenuous independent efforts of our reasoning powers the *abstract* conceptions of "moment" and "work," do we reach the satisfactory solution of the problem. "Moment" or "work" is the differentiating element. The noting of the factors "moment" or "work" having become a mental habitude, the problem no longer exists.

9.

What do we do when we abstract ?   What is an *abstraction* ?   What is a concept ?   Is there a sensuous image corresponding to every concept ?   I cannot represent to myself a general man.   I can at most represent to myself a particular man, or perhaps one combining such accidental peculiarities of different men as are not exclusive of each other.   A general triangle, which is at once right-angled and equilateral, cannot be imagined. Further, the *image* thus rising into consciousness at the *name* of the concept, and accompanying the conceptual process, is not the concept. In fact, generally, *words*, being designations which from necessity must be used to describe many different percepts, are far from being identical with concepts. A child who has seen for the first time a black dog and heard it named, soon afterward calls a large and swiftly-running black beetle, "dog"; or a pig or a sheep, "dog."[1] Any similarity whatever reminding him of the first-named percept naturally leads to the use of its name. The point of similarity need not be at all the same in the successive cases. It may reside, for instance, in one case in the color, again in the motion, then in the form, then in the external covering; and so on. Of a *concept* there is no question. Thus, a child calls the feathers of a bird "hairs"; the horns of a cow "feelers"; a brush, the beard of its father, and the down of a dandelion, without distinction, a "brush"; and so on.[2] Most adults treat words in the same manner, only less noticeably so, because they have a larger vocabulary at their disposal. The illiterate man calls a rectangle a square, and occasionally, too, a cube, a square, because of its rectangular boundaries. The science of language, and

[1] Thus the Marcomanni called the lions sent across the Danube by the Romans "dogs," and the Ionians called the χάμψαι of the Nile from the lizards of their native underbrush, "crocodiles." (Herodotus, II., 69.)

[2] All these examples are taken from experience.

a number of authenticated historical examples, show
that even nations do not act differently.[1]

A concept is never a *finished* percept.   In using a
word denoting a concept, there is nothing involved in
the word but a simple *impulse* to perform some familiar *sensory operation*, as the *result* of which a definite sensuous element (the mark of the concept) is
obtained.   For example, when I think of the concept
"heptagon," I enumerate the angles of a figure visi-
bly before me or of its image in my consciousness;
and when in so doing I reach *seven*, in which case the
sound, the numeral, or my finger announces the sensuous mark, then by this very act the given percept falls
under the given concept.   In speaking of a "square
number," I seek to resolve the number given into
components typified by the operation 5×5, 6×6, etc.,
the sensuous characteristic of which, being the *equality* of the two factors multiplied, is patent.   The same
holds good of every concept.   The sensuous activity
excited by the word may be made up of a number
of operations, one of which may involve the other.
But the result is always a *sensuous* element not *before*
present.

In looking at or in imagining a heptagon, the fact
of its having seven angles need not be present to my
mind.   This fact is distinctly cognised only on counting.   Frequently, the new sensuous element may be
so obvious (as it is, for instance, in the case of the

[1] See Whitney, *Life and Growth of Language.*

triangle) that the operation of counting seems unnecessary. Such cases, however, are exceptional, and
constitute the main source of misunderstandings concerning the nature of concepts. I do not directly *see*,
by an act of sight, in the case of conic sections (the
ellipse, parabola, hyperbola) that these curves may
be all subsumed under the same concept; but I can
discover the fact by cutting a cone, and by construct-
ing the equation for conics.

When, therefore, we apply abstract concepts to a
fact, the fact merely acts upon us as an impulse to perform a definite operation of the senses, which operation introduces *new* sensuous elements, determining
the subsequent course of our thought with reference
to the fact. By this activity we enrich and extend the
fact, which before was too meagre for us. We do
what the chemist does with his colorless solution of
salts, when by a given operation he obtains from it a
yellow or brown precipitate, having the power to dif-
ferentiate the career of his thought. The concept of
the physicist is a precise and definite *reaction-activity*,
which enriches a fact with new sensuous elements.

10.

To revert to an earlier example, when we behold
a lever, we are impelled to measure the length of
its arms, to weigh its weights, and to multiply the
numbers representing the lengths of its arms by the
numbers representing the values of its weights. If

the same sensuous numerical symbol corresponds to both products, we expect equilibrium. We have here gained a new sensuous element which was not antecedently given in the bare fact itself, but which now differentiates the career of our thought. If we will keep well in mind that thought by concepts is a reaction-activity which must be thoroughly practised, we shall understand the well-known fact that no one can familiarise himself with mathematics or physics or with any natural science by mere reading without practical exercise. Comprehension here depends entirely on action. In fact, it is impossible in any province to grasp the higher abstractions without a practical working knowledge of its details.

Facts then are extended and enriched, and ultimately again *simplified* by the action of concepts. For, when the new determinative sensuous element is found (say, the number representing the virtual moments of the lever), then this alone is investigated, and the most diverse groups of facts are found to resemble and not to resemble each other solely by virtue of this element. Thus here also, as in the case of intuitive knowledge above mentioned, everything is reducible to the discovery, selection, and emphasis of the determinative sensuous elements. Investigation here only reaches by a roundabout way what is immediately presented to intuitive cognition.

The chemist with his reactions, the physicist with his measuring rod, scales, and galvanometer, and the mathematician, all treat facts in quite the same way; the only difference being that the latter needs to go *least* outside of the elements $\alpha\beta\gamma \ldots KLM$ in his extension of facts. The aids of the mathematician are always conveniently at hand. The investigator and all his thought are a fragment only of nature, like everything else. A real chasm between him and other parts does not exist. All elements are equivalent.

On the preceding theory, the essence of abstraction is not exhausted by terming it (with Kant) *negative* attention. It is true that, in abstracting, the attention *is* turned *away* from many sensuous elements, but on the other hand, it is turned *toward* other and *new* sensuous elements; and precisely this latter fact is the essential feature. Every abstraction is founded on the prominence given to certain sensuous elements.

II.

The facts given by the senses, therefore, are alike the starting-point and the goal of all the mental adaptations of the physicist. The thoughts which follow the sense-given fact immediately are the most familiar, the strongest, and the most intuitive. Where we cannot at once follow a new fact, the strongest and most familiar thoughts press forward to lend to it their richer and preciser moulds. This process is the source of every hypothesis and speculation in science, which latter all find their warrant in the mental adaptation that has developed and ultimately given them birth.   Thus we think of the planets as projectiles, figure to ourselves an electric body as covered with a fluid that acts at a distance, think of heat as a substance that passes from one body to another, until finally the new facts become as familiar and as intuitive as the older ones, which we had used as mental helps.   Even where immediate intuition is out of the question, the thoughts of the physicist, by carefully observing the principle of *continuity* and of *sufficient differentiation*, become ordered in an economically assorted system of conceptual reactions, which lead, at least by the *shortest* path, to intuitive knowledge.

12.

Let us now consider the *results* of mental adaptation.   Thoughts can adapt themselves only to what is *constant* in the facts; the *mental reconstruction of constant elements* alone can yield advantage in point of economy.   Herein is contained the ultimate ground of our effort for *continuity* in thought, that is, for the preservation of the greatest possible constancy, and by it, too, the results of the adaptation are rendered intelligible.[1]

13.

The unconditionally constant we term *substance*. I see a body upon turning my eyes in its direction.   I can see it without touching it, I can touch it without

[1] Compare my *Mechanics*, Eng. trans., Chicago, 1893, p. 504.

seeing it. Although thus the actual appearance of the
component elements of the complex is joined to conditions, I yet have these conditions too absolutely in
my hands to appreciate or notice them markedly. I
regard the body, or the complex of elements, or the
nucleus of this complex, as always present, whether,
for the moment, it is the object of my senses or not.
Having always ready the thought of this complex, or,
symbolically, the thought of its nucleus, I gain the
advantage of being able to predict, and avoid the disadvantage of ever being surprised. My behavior is
the same with regard to the chemical elements, which
also appear to me unconditionally constant. Although
here my mere willing it is not sufficient to make of the
complexes in question sensuous facts, and although in
the present case *outward* aids also are necessary, I
yet leave these aids out of account as soon as they
have become familiar to me, and look upon the chemical elements throughout as constant. The man who
believes in atoms does the same with these auxiliary
notions.

In the same manner as with the complex of elements corresponding to a *body*, we may also proceed,
on a higher plane of thought-adaptation, with entire
provinces of facts. In speaking of electricity, magnetism, light, and heat, even when not associating
substances with these names, we yet ascribe constancy
to these provinces of facts, leaving entirely out of account the *familiar conditions* under which they ap-

pear; and we hold the ideas which reproduce them
always in readiness, thereby gaining an advantage
similar to that explained above.   When I say a body
is "electric," far more memories arise in my mind,
and my expectations are associated with far more
definite groups of facts, than if I had emphasised, for
instance, the attractions displayed in the single cases.
Yet this hypostasising may have its disadvantages, also.
In the first place, in proceeding thus, we always follow
the same historical paths. It may be important, however, to recognise that there is no such thing as a specific *electrical* fact, that every such fact can just as
well be regarded, for example, as a chemical one, or
as a thermal one, or rather that all physical facts are
made up, in an ultimate analysis, of the same sensuous elements (colors, pressures, spaces, times), and
that we are merely reminded by the term "electric"
of that particular form in which we first became acquainted with the fact.

If we have once accustomed ourselves to regard
the body, to and from which we can, at pleasure, turn
our glance and touching hand, as constant, then it is
easy for us to do the same in cases in which the conditions of sensuous manifestation lie entirely without
our reach—for example, in the case of the sun and
moon, which we cannot touch, or of parts of the world
which we have seen but once and shall perhaps never
see again, or that we know only by description. Such
a method of procedure may have a high importance

in an undisturbed and economical conception of the world, but it is certainly not the only legitimate method. It would be merely a consistent additional step, if we were to regard the whole past, which is, indeed, still present in its vestiges (since, for instance, we see the stars where they were thousands of years ago) and the whole future, which is present in germ (since, for example, our solar system will be seen where it now is, thousands of years hence) as constant. The entire *passage of time*, in fact, is dependent solely on conditions of sensuous activity. Were a special purpose given, even this step might be hazarded.

14.

Really unconditioned constancy does not exist, as will be evident from the preceding considerations. We attain to the idea of absolute constancy only as we overlook or underrate conditions, or as we regard them as always given, or as we deliberately *disregard* them. There is but one sort of constancy, which embraces all forms, namely, constancy of *connexion* (or of *relation*).

The majority of the propositions of natural science express such constancies of connexion : "The tadpole is metamorphosed into a frog; chlorate of sodium makes its appearance in the form of cubes. Rays of light are rectilinear. Bodies fall with an acceleration of 9.81 (*m/sec* ^{2})." When these constancies are expressed in concepts, we call them laws. Force (in the mechanical signification) is likewise merely a constancy of connexion. When I say that a body A exerts a force on a body B, I mean that B, on coming into contraposition with A, is immediately affected by a certain acceleration with respect to A.

The singular illusion, that the substance A is the *absolutely constant vehicle* of a *force* which takes effect immediately on B's being contraposed to A, is easily shattered. If we, or more exactly speaking, our sense-organs, be put in the place of B, here a *condition* intervenes, which, seeing that it is possible at any time to fulfil it, is invariably disregarded, and thus A appears to us absolutely constant. Similarly, a magnet, which we see as often as we care to look in its direction, appears to us the constant vehicle of a magnetic force, which becomes operative only upon being brought near to a particle of iron, which we cannot disregard as easily as ourselves without noticing the fact.[1] The phrases, "No matter without force, no force without matter," which are but abortive attempts to remove a self-incurred contradiction, become superfluous on our recognising only *constancies* of *connexion.*

[1] To the child everything appears substantial, for perceiving which only his senses are necessary. The child asks where the shadow, where the extinguished light goes to. He will not suffer the electrical machine to be turned any great length of time for fear of exhausting the supply of sparks, etc.—Only upon noting conditions of a fact that are *outside* ourselves does the impression of substantiality disappear. The history of the theory of heat is very instructive in this connexion.

15.

Given a sufficient constancy of environment, there is developed a corresponding constancy of thought. By virtue of this constancy our thoughts are spontaneously impelled to *complete* all incompletely observed facts. The impulse in question is not prompted by the individual facts as observed at the time ; nor is it intentionally evoked ; but we find it operative in ourselves entirely without our personal intervention. It confronts us like a power *from without,* yet as a power which continually accompanies and assists us, as a thing of which we stand in need, in order to supply the deficiencies of the fact. Although it is developed by experience, it contains *more* than is contained in the single experience. The impulse in a certain measure *enriches* the single fact. Through it the latter is *more* to us. By this impulse we have always a *larger* portion of nature in our field of vision than the inexperienced man has, with the single fact alone. For the human being, with his thoughts and his impulses, is himself merely a piece of nature, which is added to the single fact. This impulse, however, can lay no claim to infallibility, and there exists no necessity compelling the facts to correspond to it. Our confidence in it rests entirely upon the supposition, which has been substantiated by numerous trials, of the sufficiency of the mental adaptation,—a supposition, however, which must be prepared to be contradicted at any moment.

Not all our ideas representing facts have the same constancy. Whenever we have a special interest in the representation of facts, we endeavor to support and corroborate ideas of lesser constancy by ideas of greater constancy, or to replace them by the latter. Thus Newton conceived the planets as projectiles, although Kepler's laws were already well known, the tides as attracted by the moon, although the facts of their movement had long been ascertained. We believe we understand the suction of a pump, the flowing of a siphon, only as we add in thought the pressure of the air. Similarly we seek to conceive electrical, optical, and thermal processes as *mechanical* processes. This need of the support of weaker thoughts by stronger thoughts is also called the *need of causality*, and is the moving spring of all explanation in science. We naturally prefer, as the foundation of this process, the strongest and most thoroughly tested thoughts, and these are given us by our much exercised mechanical functions, which we may test anew at any moment without many or cumbersome appliances. Hence the authority of mechanical explanations, especially those by pressure and impact. A corresponding and still higher authority attaches to mathematical thoughts, for in their development we stand in need of no extraneous means whatever, but on the contrary, invariably carry most of the material for experimenting about with us. But if we are once apprised of this, the need of mechanical explanations is appreciably weakened.[1]

It was said above that man himself is a fragment of nature. Let me illustrate this by an example. For the chemist a substance may be sufficiently character- ised merely by his sensations. In this case the chem- ist *himself* supplies, by *inner* means, the whole wealth of fact necessary to the determination of his course of thought. But in other cases, resources to reaction by the help of *outward* means may be necessary. When an electric current flows round a magnetic needle situ- ated in its plane, the north pole of the needle is de- flected to my left if I imagine myself as Ampère's swimmer in the current. I enrich the fact (current and needle) which is insufficient in itself to define the direction of my thought, by introducing *myself* into the experiment by an inner reaction. I may like- wise lay my watch in the plane of the circuit, so that the hand moves in the direction of the current. Then the south pole falls in front of, the north pole behind the dial. Or I may make of the circuit traversed by the current a sun-dial (on the plan of which the watch

[1] Physical experiences other than mechanical may approach to the value of mechanical experiences as they become more familiar. In my opinion Stricker has advanced a correct and important view in bringing causality into connexion with the will. When I was a young docent, I myself advocated with great warmth and onesidedness (in the exposition of Mill's method of difference) the view expressed by Stricker. And the idea has never quite left me (comp., for example, my *Science of Mechanics*, Eng. trans., pp. 84, 304, 485.) However, I am at present of the opinion, as the above discussion shows, that this question is not so simple and must be looked at from *several* sides.

in fact was modelled), so arranging it that the shadow follows the current. In this case the north pole will move towards the shadowed side of the plane of the current. The two last-mentioned reactions are *outward* reactions. The two species of reactions could not be made use of indiscriminately if a chasm existed between myself and the world. Nature is a single whole. The fact that the two species of reaction are not known in all cases, and that frequently the observer appears to be entirely without influence, proves nothing against the view advanced.

16.

Whenever it happens, in a complexus of elements, that some of the elements get replaced by others, necessarily the constancy of the connexion is *changed.* In such cases it is desirable to discover a constancy which survives this change. J. R. Mayer first felt this need, and satisfied it by enunciating his concept of "force," which corresponds to the technical mechanical concept of "work" (Poncelet) or more exactly to the more general concept of "energy." Mayer conceives this force (or energy) as something absolutely constant (as a store of something, as a substance), and so goes back to the strongest and most intuitive thoughts. We perceive, from Mayer's struggle with expressions, with general philosophical phrases, etc. (noticeable in the first and second of his treatises), that he at first felt *instinctively* and *intuitively* the urgent need of such a concept. But the great achievement was accomplished only upon his *adapting* the existing physical concepts to the requirements of the facts *and* his needs.[1]

[1] In observing a freely falling body, we note the constancy $v=\sqrt{2gh}$, which we may also, if we like, express in the form $gh=v^2/2$. Making the entire possible distance of descent $H=h+h'$, then also $gh'+v^2/2 = const.$ We may now imagine a *constant* stock of something (figuratively a substance) which, when the event occurs, is converted from the form gh' into the form $v^2/2$, or if $ph'+mv^2/2$ be made constant, from the form ph' into the form $mv^2/2$, but which always preserves its total value unchanged. Such a conception is well qualified to meet our *needs* and to turn our thoughts into familiar channels. Nevertheless, there is nothing compelling us to regard gh and $v^2/2$ as equivalent. In the first equation $v=\sqrt{2gh}$, there is no perceptible trace of such a conception. If it be found, however, that when $mv^2/2$ disappears ph' may reappear (for instance, in the rebound of an elastic ball), then this conception serves a highly practical purpose. (Comp. Mach, *Erhaltung der Arbeit*, p. 45, and for many instructive discussions of particulars, the admirable work of J. Popper, *Die physikalischen Grundsätze der electrischen Kraftübertragung.*)

If the body does not fall freely, but in gradually sinking heats another body or renders it electric, then an entirely new constancy takes the place of the first. Nothing compels us to regard the quantity of heat generated or the electric potential produced as the equivalent of the missing $mv^2/2$. Our determining that the heat *shall stand for exactly as much as* the corresponding ph' is *arbitrary*, notwithstanding its great convenience. It was primarily Mayer's *need* that led him to write down his equation, which as regards the facts was not as yet satisfied and which is generally incorrect if the right units are not selected.

Facts can teach us constancy of connexion only. In *reversible* processes (processes that are independent of time) we find *periodic* changes of elements connected with *periodic* changes of other elements, simply. There is nothing in this of equivalence. Heat may take the place of ph', and in place of this again the same ph' may reappear. This gives the conception *practical* value. With reference to changes which are not reversible (changes dependent on time) the conception of equivalence is idle. Whether or not heat which can no longer reappear as work may still be regarded as the equivalent of work, is of no consequence. We might be struck by the *proportionality* between ph and *quantity* of heat, and think that this certainly could not depend upon an arbitrary conception but must inhere in nature. Yet if we had attempted, say, to regard ph and *quantity* of electricity as equivalent, this conception would have proved unserviceable, and the idea would necessarily have required modification until energy had been substituted for quantity of electricity. That *quantity* of heat was so readily offered in the inquiry, was a fortunate historical circumstance, which militates in no wise against the correctness of our considerations.—Mayer's unusually powerful intellectual in-

17.

Upon sufficient adaptation, the facts are spontaneously reproduced by the thoughts, and *incompletely*
given facts are *completed*. Physics can act only as a
quantitative norm regulating and giving a more *precise*
conformation to the spontaneously flowing thoughts,
suitably to definite practical or scientific needs. When
I see a body thrown horizontally, the vivid picture of
a projectile in motion rises before my mind. But the
artilleryman or the physicist requires more. He must
know, for example, that if on applying the measuring-
rod M to the horizontal abscissæ of the projectile's
path, he can *count* to 1, 2, 3, 4 . . . . he must, on applying the measure M' to the vertical ordinates, also
count to 1, 4, 9, 16 . . . . in order to reach a point of
the path. The function of physics consists, therefore,
in teaching that a fact which, on a *definite* reaction R
yields a sensory mark E, also yields, on the giving of
a *different* reaction R', a second sensory mark E'. By
this means it is possible to supply more exactly the
deficiencies of incompletely given facts.

stinct combined with strength of conceptual thought, his broad, comprehensive vision, the clearness with which he ultimately determined the mechanical equivalent of heat without resorting to a new experiment, characterises
him as an investigator of the first rank. But it by no means follows from
this fact, that those inquirers who came after him were dishonest. On the
contrary, I am convinced, from all the evidence accessible to me, that the
investigators in question all followed *independent* courses of reasoning,—a
conclusion that I cannot further discuss here.

18.

The space of the geometrician is by no means made up wholly of the system of space-*sensations* (of the senses of sight and touch), but consists rather of a large body of *physical* observations, having the space-sensations as their point of departure. In the very fact of the geometrician's regarding his space as constituted at all points and in all directions alike, he goes far beyond the space given by sight and touch, which by no means possesses this simple property (p. 80). Without experience in *physics* the geometrician would never have reached this conception. The fundamental propositions of geometry have, as a fact, been acquired wholly by means of physical observations, by the superposition of measures of length and of angles, by the application of *rigid* bodies to one another. Without propositions of *congruence*, no geometry. Apart from the fact that spatial images would never have been produced in us without physical experience, we should, even granting their existence, never have been able to apply them to one another and to test their congruence, without this knowledge. When we feel *compelled* to imagine an isosceles triangle as having equal angles at its base, our compulsion is due to the remembrance of powerful past experiences. If the proposition had its source in "pure intuition," there would be no necessity for learning it.[1]   That

---

[1] The method of Euclid is undoubtedly excellent for the instruction of adult persons, with abundant geometric experience. It serves to protect us

discoveries may be made by sheer power of geometrical imagination, and are made so daily, merely proves that the *memory* of a given experience can reveal to the mind features which in the original observation escaped unnoticed; just as in the after-image of a brightly-lighted lamp, new and previously unseen details may be discovered. Even the theory of numbers must be looked at in some such manner; its fundamental propositions can hardly be viewed as entirely independent of physical experience.

The cogency of geometry (and of all mathematics) is due, not to the fact that its theories are arrived at by some select and special kind of cognition, but only to the fact that the empirical material which is at its base is particularly convenient and handy, has been put to the test an untold number of times, and can be subjected again at any moment to the same tests. Moreover, the province of space-experience is far more limited than that of the whole of experience. The conviction of having essentially exhausted this limited province soon arises and produces the necessary self-confidence.

A self-confidence similar to that of the geometrician is doubtless also possessed by the composer and the decorative painter, who have both gained, the former in the domain of sensations of tone, ·the latter

from the possible errors which we have acquired. That no worse results have been entailed by use of this method in instructing the youth is due entirely to the fact that nobody comes into the hands of a teacher altogether without geometrical experience.

in that of sensations of color, a broad and rich experience. To the one no space-figure will occur the elements of which are not well known to him, and the two others will meet with no new combinations of tone or of color that are unfamiliar to them. But the inexperienced beginner in geometry will be *no less* surprised and disappointed than the young musician or decorator.

The mathematician, the composer, the decorator, and the student of natural science, when indulging in *speculative* flights, pursue quite *analogous* modes of procedure, despite the differences of their matter and aim. The former, it is true, owing to his more limited material, has the advantage of the others as regards the certainty of his procedure; while the latter for the opposite reason is at a disadvantage as compared with the others.

19.

In like manner, the *time* of the physicist does not coincide with the system of time-*sensations.* When the physicist wishes to determine a period of time, he applies, as his instruments of measurement, *identical* processes or processes *assumed to be identical,* such as vibrations of a pendulum, the rotations of the earth, etc. The fact connected with the time-sensation is in this manner made the subject of a reaction, and the result of the latter, the *number* which is obtained, serves, in place of the time-*sensation,* to determine more exactly the subsequent movement of the thought. In like manner, we regulate our thoughts concerning thermal processes not according to the *sensation* of warmth which bodies yield us, but according to the much more definite sensation which is obtained from *thermometrical reactions* by simply *noting* the height of the mercury. Usually a space-sensation (the dial of a clock) is substituted for the sensation of time, and for this, again, a *number* is put. For example, if we represent the excess of the temperature of a cooling body over that of its surroundings by $\vartheta = \Theta_e^{-kt}$, then *t* is this number.

The relation which the quantities of an equation actually represent, is usually (analytically) a more general one than that which is meant to be represented by the equation. Thus in the equation $(x/a)^2 + (y/b)^2 = 1$ all possible values of *x* have an *analytical* meaning, and yield corresponding values of $\dot{y}$. But if the equation be used to represent an ellipse, then only the values of $x < a$ and $y < b$ have a *geometrical* (or real) significance.

Similarly, it would have to be expressly added, if this were not obvious, that the equation $\vartheta = \Theta_e^{-kt}$ represents the real process only for *increasing* values of *t*.

If we imagine the natural course of different events, say the cooling of one body and the free descent of a second, represented by equations involving time, the time may be eliminated from these equations, and we may express, for example, the space traversed by the falling body in terms of the excess of temperature. Thus viewed, the elements appear simply as dependent on *one another*. But the meaning of such an equation must be more exactly defined by premising that only *increasing* distances of descent or *decreasing* temperatures are to be inserted successively therein.

Time is not *reversible*. A warm body set in cool surroundings simply cools off but does not grow warm again. With increasing time-sensations only decreasing excesses of temperature are connected. A house in flames burns down but never builds itself up again. A plant does not decrease in size and creep into the earth, but grows out of it, increasing in size. The irreversibility of time reduces itself to the fact that the value-changes of physical quantities always take place in *definite directions*. Of the two analytical possibilities one only is *actual*. We do not need to see in this fact a metaphysical problem.

APPENDIX I.

FACTS AND MENTAL SYMBOLS.[1]

I PURSUED in my youth physical *and* philosophical studies, particularly psychology, with equal ardor. At that time there was hardly a question of an experimental psychology, of a relation of psychological to physiological research. Neither did the physics of that day think of a psychological analysis of the notions it was constantly employing. How the notions of "body," "matter," "atom," etc., originated, was not investigated. Objects were given the inviolability of which physicists never questioned and with which they unconcernedly pursued their labors.

The fields of physical and psychological research thus stood side by side *unreconciled*, each having its own particular concepts, methods, and theories. No one doubted that the two departments were in some

---

[1] Written in 1891, and published in *The Monist* of January, 1892 (Vol. II., No. 2), in continuation of the discussion with Dr. Paul Carus in Vol. I., No. 3 of *The Monist* on "Some Questions of Psycho-physics." The few controversial references are omitted. Professor Mach is explaining the grounds which led him to abandon his early position, that Nature has two sides, a physical and a psychological, which view he likens to that held by the editor of *The Monist.—Trans.*

way connected.   But the nature of the connexion appeared an insoluble riddle, as it still appears to Dubois-Reymond.

Now although this condition of things was not such as to satisfy my mind, it was nevertheless natural that as a student I should seek to acquire tentatively the dominant views of the two provinces and to put them into consistent connexion with one another.

I thus formed provisorily the view that Nature has two *sides*—a physical and a psychological side.   If psychical life is to be harmonised at all with the theories of physics, we are obliged, I reasoned, to conceive of atoms as *feeling* (ensouled).   The various dynamic phenomena of the atoms would then represent the physical processes, whilst the internal states *connected therewith* would be the phenomena of psychic life.   If we accept in faith and seriousness the atomistic speculations of the physicists and of the early psychologists (on the unity of the soul), I still see no other way of arriving at a tenable monistic conception.

It is unnecessary to emphasise at length here the prominent part which the artificial scaffolding employed in the construction of knowledge plays in these monadic theories as contradistinguished from the facts which really deserve to be known, and the scant satisfaction which such theories afford in the long run.   As a fact, employment with this cumbrous artifice was in my case the very means that gave rise to my better conviction, which was already latently present.[1]

In the further progress of my physical work I soon discovered that it was very necessary *sharply to distinguish* between what we *see* and what we mentally *supply*. When, for example, I imagine heat as a substance (a fluid) that passes from one body to another, I follow with ease the phenomena of conduction and

[1] A Greek philosopher to whom change of spatial configuration, pressure, and impact were probably the only natural processes with which he was intimately acquainted, thought out the atomistic theory. This theory we retain to-day, though in a modified form. And in fact natural phenomena really do exist such that, to all appearances, the pressure and impact of very small particles are concerned in their production (the dynamical theory of gases), phenomena that therefore admit of being more clearly viewed by this conception. However, this conception, like that of caloric, possesses value only in certain fields. We know to-day that pressure and impact are by no means simpler phenomena than are for example the phenomena of gravitation. The contention that in physics everything can be reduced to the motion of smallest particles is, at best, but an improper draft on the future. Utterances of this kind afford no assistance in the solution of burning special questions, but only confound, and have about the same explanatory value as the utterances of the late physical philosophy of Oken,—a philosophy which, for example, reproduces with the greatest ease the method of the creation of the world by a division of zero-quantities into $+a$ and $-a$ ($0 = +a - a$).

The motion of a *single* body as a totality does indeed appear simpler at first glance than any other process, and this is the justification of attempts at a *physical* monadic theory. The thoughts of a *single* man are connected together; the thoughts of two different men are not. How can the processes of the different parts of the brain of one man be connected? In order to make the connexion very intimate, we conceive everything that requires to be psychically connected, as collected in *a single* point, although the connexion is not explained by our procedure. Thus the psychological monadic theory rests on a motive and on an illusion quite similar to those on which the physical rests.

Let us assume for a moment the proposition in the text; viz., that the atoms are endowed with feeling. By the space-coördinates $x, y, z, x', y', z' \ldots$ of the atoms are determined *in the atoms* internal conditions $a, \beta, \gamma, a', \beta', \gamma' \ldots$, and *vice versa*. For we feel by our senses our physical environment, and our reactions upon our environment are conditioned by our sensations. The idea then suggests itself, since $a \beta \gamma \ldots$ alone are directly given, to set up by the elimination of $x, y, z \ldots$ equations directly between $a \beta \gamma, a' \beta' \gamma' \ldots$. This view would very nearly approach to my present one, (apart from the fact that the latter entirely rejects metaphysical considerations).

exchange. This idea led Black, who established it, to the discovery of specific heat, of the latent heat of fusion and vaporisation, and so forth. *This same* idea of a constant quantity of heat-substance, on the other hand, *prevented* Black's successors from using their eyes. They no longer observe the fact which every savage knows, that heat is *produced* by friction. By the help of his undulatory theory Huygens follows with ease the phenomena of luminous reflexion and refraction. The same theory *prevents* him (for he thinks solely of the longitudinal waves with which he is familiar), from rightly grasping the fact of polarisation which he himself discovered, but which Newton, on the other hand, untrammelled by theories, perceives at once. The conception of fluids acting at a distance on conductors charged with electricity facilitates our view of the behavior of the objects charged, but it *stood in the way of* the discovery of the specific inductive capacity, which was reserved for the eye of Faraday undimmed by traditional conceptions.

Valuable, therefore, as are the conceptions which we mentally (theoretically) supply in investigating facts, bringing to bear, as they do, older, richer, more general, and more familiar experiences on facts that stand alone, thus affording us a broader field of view, nevertheless, the same conceptions may lead us astray as classical examples and our own experience demonstrate. For a theory, indeed, always puts in the place of a fact something *different*, something more simple,

which is qualified to represent the fact in some *certain*
aspect, but for the very reason that it is different does
not represent it in other aspects.   When in the place
of *light* Huygens mentally put the familiar phenomenon of *sound*, light itself appeared to him as a thing
that he knew, but with respect to polarisation, which
sound-waves lack, as a thing with which he was doubly
unacquainted.   Our theories are abstractions, which,
while placing in relief what is important in *certain
determinate* cases, neglect almost necessarily, or even
disguise, what is important in other cases.   The law
of refraction looks upon rays of light as homogeneous
straight lines, and that is sufficient for the comprehension of the geometrical aspect of the matter.   But the
propositions relating to refraction will never lead us
to the fact that the rays of light are periodical, that
they interfere.   On the contrary, the favorite and
familiar conception of a ray as an undifferentiated
straight line is more likely to render this discovery
difficult.

The instances in which the resemblance between a
fact and its theoretical conception extends *further* than
we ourselves postulate, are rare.   But when this happens, the theoretical conception may lead to the discovery of *new* facts, a case of which conical refraction,
circular polarisation, and Hertz's electric waves furnish
examples that militate against those above advanced.
As a general rule, however, there is every reason for
distinguishing sharply between our theoretical con-

ceptions of phenomena and that which we observe. The former must be regarded merely as auxiliary instruments which have been created for a *definite* purpose and which possess permanent value only with respect to that purpose. No serious person will imagine for a moment that real circles with angles and sines perform functions in the refraction of light. Every one, on the contrary, regards the formula $\sin\alpha/\sin\beta = n$ as a kind of geometrical model which simply *imitates in form* the refraction of light and *takes its place* in our mind. Now, in this sense, I take it, all theoretical conceptions of physics—caloric, electricity, light-waves, molecules, atoms, and energy—must be regarded as mere helps or expedients to facilitate our consideration of things. Even within the domain of physics itself the greatest care must be exercised in transferring theories from one department to another, and above all more information is not to be expected from a theory than from the facts themselves.

On the other hand, there is no lack of instances showing the far greater confusion which was produced by the direct transference of theories, methods, and inquiries that were legitimate in physics, into the field of psychology.

Allow me to illustrate this by a few examples.

A physicist observes an image on the retina of an excised eye, notices that it is turned upside down with respect to the objects imaged, and puts to himself

very naturally the question, How does a luminous
point situated *at the top* come to be reflected on the
retina *at the bottom ?* He answers this question by the
aid of studies in dioptrics. If, now, this question,
which is perfectly legitimate in the province of physics, be transferred to the domain of psychology, only
obscurity will be produced. The question why we see
the *inverted* retinal image *upright*, has no meaning as
a psychological problem. The light-sensations of the
separate spots of the retina are connected with sensations of locality from the very outset, and we *name* the
places that correspond to the parts down, *up*. To the
perceiving subject such a question cannot present itself.

It is the same with the well-known theory of projection. The problem of the *physicist* is, to seek the
luminous object-point of a point imaged on the retina
of the eye, in the backward prolonged ray passing
through the centre of the eye. For the perceiving
subject this *problem* does not exist, as the light-sensations of the retinal spots are connected from the beginning with determinate space-sensations. The entire theory of the psychological origin of the "external"
world by the projection of sensations outwards is
founded in my opinion on a mistaken transference of
a *physically* formulated inquiry into the province of
psychology. Our sensations of sight and touch are
bound up with, are connected with, various *different*
sensations of space, that is to say, the sensations in

question have an existence *by the side of* one another or *outside of* one another, exist, in other words, in a *spatial* field, in which our body fills but a part.   That table is thus self-evidently *outside* of my body.   A projection-problem does not present itself, is neither con· sciously nor unconsciously solved.

A physicist (Mariotte) discovers that a certain spot on the retina is blind.   He is accustomed to associating with every spatial point an imaged point, and with every imaged point a sensation.   Hence the question arises, What do we see at the points corresponding to the blind spots, and how is the gap in the image filled out ?   If the unfounded influence of the physicist's methods on the discussion of psychological questions be excluded, it will be found that no problem exists at all here.   We see *nothing* at the blind spots, the gap in the image is *not* filled out.   The gap, furthermore, is not felt, for the reason that a defect of light-sensation at a spot blind from the beginning can no more be perceived as a gap in the image than the blindness say of the skin of the back can be so perceived.

I have intentionally chosen simple and obvious examples, as they can best render clear what unnecessary confusion is caused by the careless transference of a conception or mode of thought which is valid and serviceable in one domain, into another.

In the work of a celebrated German ethnographer I recently read the following sentence : "This tribe of people deeply degraded itself by the practice of

cannibalism." By its side lay the book of an English inquirer who deals with the same subject. The
latter simply puts the question *why* certain South-Sea
Islanders eat human beings, finds out in the course of
his inquiries that our own ancestors were once cannibals, and comes to understand the position the Hindus
take in the matter --a point of view that occurred once
to my five year-old boy who while eating a piece of
meat stopped, suddenly shocked, and cried out, "*We*
are cannibals to the animals !" "Thou shalt not eat
human beings" is a very beautiful maxim ; but in the
mouth of the ethnographer it sullies the calm and
noble lustre of unprepossession by which we so gladly
discover the true inquirer.   But a step further and we
shall say, "Man *must* not be descended from monkeys," "The earth *shall* not rotate," "Matter *ought*
not everywhere to fill space," "Energy *must* be constant," and so on. I believe that our procedure differs
from that just characterised only in degree and not in
kind, when we transfer views reached in the province
of physics, with the dictum of sovereign validity, into
the domain of psychology, where they should be tested
anew with respect to their serviceability.   In such
cases we are subject to dogma, if not to dogma which
is forced upon us by a power from without like our
scholastic forefathers, yet to that which we have created ourselves.   And what result of research is there
that could not become a dogma by long habit and use,
since the very skill which we have acquired in familiar

intellectual situations deprives us of the freshness and unprepossession which are so requisite in the new!

Now that I have set forth in general outlines the position I take, I may perhaps be able to explain my opposition to the *dualism of feeling and motion.* This dualism is to my mind artificial and unnecessary. Its origin is analogous to that of certain pseudo-mathematical problems,—having come from an improper formulation of the questions involved.

In the investigation of purely physical processes we generally employ concepts of so abstract a character that as a rule we think only cursorily, or not at all, of the sensations that lie at their base. For example, when I ascertain the fact that an electric current having the strength of 1 Ampère develops $10\frac{1}{2}$ cubic centimetres of oxyhydrogen gas at 0° C. and 760 mm mercury-pressure in a minute, I am readily disposed to attribute to the objects defined a reality wholly independent of my sensations. But I am obliged, in order to arrive at what I have determined, to conduct the current through a circular wire having a definite measured radius, so that the current, the intensity of terrestrial magnetism being given, shall turn the magnetic needle at its centre a certain angular distance out of the meridian. The intensity of terrestrial magnetism must have been disclosed by a definite observed period of vibration of a magnetic needle of measured dimensions, known weight, and so forth. The determination of the oxyhydrogen gas

is no less intricate.   The whole statement, so simple
in its appearance, is based upon an almost unending
series of simple sensory observations (sensations), particularly if we take into consideration the observations
that assure the adjustment of the apparatus, which
may have been performed in part long before the actual experiment.   Now it can easily happen to the
physicist who does not study the psychology of his
operations, that he does not (to reverse a well-known
saying) see the trees for the woods, that he slurs over
the sensory elements at the foundation of his work.
Now I maintain that every physical concept is nothing
but a certain definite connexion of the sensory *elements*
which I denote by $A B C . . .$, and that every physical
fact rests therefore on such a connexion.   These *elements*—elements in the sense that no further resolu-
tion has as yet been made of them—are the simplest
building-stones of the physical world that we have yet
been able to reach.

Physiological research also may be of a purely
physical character.   I can follow the course of a physical process as it propagates itself through a sensitive
nerve to the spinal cord and brain of an animal and returns by various paths to the muscles, whose contraction produces further effects in the environment of
the animal.   I need not think, in so doing, of any feeling on the part of the animal; what I investigate is a
purely physical object.   Very much is lacking, it is
true, to our complete comprehension of the details of

this process, and the assurance that it is all *motion* can neither console me nor deceive me with respect to my ignorance.

Long prior to scientific psychology people had perceived that the behavior of an animal confronted by physical influences is much better grasped, that is understood, by attributing to the animal *sensations* like our own. To that which I see, to *my* sensations, I have to *supply mentally* the sensations of the *animal,* which are not to be found in the province of my own sensation. This opposition appears even more abrupt to the scientific inquirer who is investigating a nervous process by the aid of colorless abstract concepts, and is required for example to add mentally to that process the sensation green. This last may actually appear as something entirely novel, and we may ask ourselves how it is that this miraculous thing is produced from chemical processes, electrical currents, and the like.[1]

Psychological analysis has taught us that this surprise is unjustifiable, since the physicist deals with

[1] The following is a legitimate question: To what kind of nervous processes is the sensation green to be mentally added? Such questions can be solved only by special inquiry, and not by reference in a general way to motion and electric currents. How disadvantageous it is for us to remain satisfied with such general conceptions can be seen from the fact that inquirers have been repeatedly on the brink of abandoning the *specific energies*, one of the greatest acquisitions we have made, simply because they were unable to discover any difference in the currents of different sensory nerves. I was impelled as early as 1863 in my lectures on psycho-physics to call attention to the fact that the *most diverse kinds* of nervous processes can conceal themselves in a current. Current is an abstraction and places in relief but one feature of the process—the passage of energy through a transverse section. A current in diluted sulphuric acid is something entirely different from a current in copper. We must therefore expect also that a current in the acoustic nerve will be something entirely different from a current in the optic nerve.

sensations in all his work. The same analysis may also show us that the mental addition by analogy of sensations and complexes of sensations which at the time being are not present in the field of sense or cannot even come into it, is daily practised by the physicist, as, for example, when he imagines the moon an inert heavy mass, although he cannot touch the moon but can only see it. The totally strange character of the intellectual situation above described is therefore an illusion.

The illusion disappears when I make observations (psychologically) on my own person, which are limited to the sensory sphere. Before me lies the leaf of a plant. The green (A) of the leaf is united with a certain optical sensation of space (B) and sensation of touch (C), and with the visibility of the sun or the lamp (D). If the yellow (E) of a sodium flame takes the place of the sun, the green (A) will pass into brown (F). If the chlorophyl granules be removed,— an operation representable, like the preceding one, by elements,—the green (A) will pass into white (G). All these observations are *physical* observations. But the green (A) is also united with a certain process on my retina. There is nothing to prevent me in principle from physically investigating this process in my own eye in exactly the same manner as in the cases previously set forth, and from reducing it to its elements $X\ Y\ Z$. . . . If this were not possible in the case of my own eye, it might be accomplished with that of another, and the gap filled out by analogy, exactly as in physical investigations. Now in its dependence upon *B C D*. . . ., *A* is a *physical element*, in its dependence on *X Y Z* . . . it is a *sensation*. The green (*A*), however, is not altered at all *in itself*, whether we direct our attention to the one or to the other form of dependence. *I see, therefore, no opposition of physical and psychical, no duality, but simply identity.* In the sensory sphere of my consciousness everything is at once physical and psychical.

The obscurity of this intellectual situation has, I take it, arisen solely from the transference of a physical prepossession to the domain of psychology. The physicist says : I find everywhere bodies and the motions of bodies only, no sensations ; sensations, therefore, must be something *entirely different* from the physical objects I deal with. The psychologist accepts the second portion of this declaration. To him, it is true, sensation is *given*, but there corresponds to it a mysterious physical something which conformably to physical prepossession must be *different* from sensation. But what is it that is the really mysterious thing ? Is it the Physis or the Psyche ? Or is it perhaps *both ?* It would almost appear so, as it is now the one and now the other that is intangible. Or does the whole argument rest on a vicious circle ?

I believe that the latter is the case. For me the elements designated by *A B C* . . . are immediately and indubitably given, and for me they can never afterwards be volatilised away by considerations which ultimately are always based on their existence.[1]

For that department of special research having for its subject the sensory, physical, and psychical province which is not made superfluous by this general orientation and which cannot be forestalled, only the relations of A B C . . . remain to be ascertained. This may be expressed symbolically by saying that it is the purpose and end of special research to find equations of the form $f(A, B, C . . .) = 0$.

*   *   *

This whole train of reasoning has for me simply the significance of negative orientation for the avoidance of pseudo-problems. Moreover, I intentionally restrict myself here to the question of sense-perceptions, for the reason that at the start exact special research will find here alone a safe basis of operations.

---

[1] It is the transitoriness of sense-perceptions that so easily leads us to regard them as mere appearances in contrast with permanent bodies. I have repeatedly pointed out that *unconditioned* permanent things do not exist in nature, that permanences of connexion only exist. A body is for me the same complex of sight-and-touch-sensations every time that it is placed in the same circumstances of illumination, position in space, temperature, and so forth. The supposed constancy of the body is the constancy of the union of A B C . . . or the constancy of the *equation* $f(A, B, C . . .) = 0$.

APPENDIX II.

A NEW ACOUSTIC EXPERIMENT BY E. MACH.[1]

IN A box having double walls, the intervening space of which is packed with sawdust, is placed an electric tuning-fork, reed-pipe, or other musical instrument which can be easily excited from without. (See next page, Fig. 37, which is drawn from memory.) From this box runs a tube which divides into two branches. One of these branches leads to a König's manometric capsule; the other is carried close to a pasteboard disc where it breaks but on the other side is continued again to the ear of the observer. The pasteboard disc, which can be turned like the disc of an electrical machine, has a radial slit of variable angular width, and carries at the proper inclination to its axis a mirror into which the observer can look through the slit.

Exciting the apparatus in the box, and putting the eye close to the disc, which is now set in rotation, the ear receives the impression of a uniform tone, the

[1] Extract from *Lotos*, Prague, August, 1873. Reprinted to elucidate the reference on page 124.

duration of which is curtailed by the slit.   In the rotating mirror is seen the image of the manometric
gas-jet, which is resolved into distinct and single
flames, the resultant action of the slit being that the

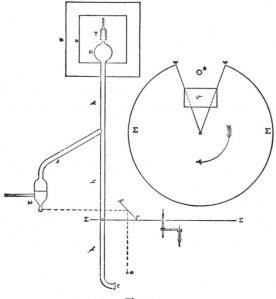

Fig. 37.

(Diagram Explaining "A New Acoustic Experiment by E. Mach."
Drawn from memory.)

T, electric tuning-fork. *BB*, box with double walls. *R*, resonator. *ttt*,
tube. *M*, Manometric capsule. *ΣΣ*, rotating disc with variable slit *WW*.
σσ, mirror attached to the disc behind the slit. *E*, the ear. *O*, the eye.

observer *sees* as many vibrations as he *hears*. We can
count thus, by enumerating the images of the flames,
the number of vibrations reaching the ear, and so convince ourselves that for the production of the sensa-

tion of *tone* a certain number of vibrations are required. If the ear receives too few vibrations no tone is noticed, but only a short, *sharp* concussion, in which no pitch is distinguishable. A low tone of one hundred and twenty-eight full vibrations is recognisable as a tone of definite pitch only upon four to five vibrations striking the ear; with two or three vibrations it produces only a sharp concussion. In the case of low tones the harmonics are distinctly heard when the fundamental, from its brief duration, is undistinguishable.

ADDENDA.

PAGE 97, LAST FOOTNOTE.—Add the words: "The same phenomena may also be observed in connexion with the shadow of the moon and of the planets (Seeliger, *Abhandlungen der Münchener Akademie*, II. Cl., XIX. Bd., II. Abtheil., 1896)."

PAGE 105.—Add as a footnote to the last line of paragraph 11: "Compare on this point Jacques Loeb, *Ueber den Nachweis von Contrasterscheinungen im Gebiete der Raumempfindungen des Auges*, *Archiv f. Physiologie*, Bd. 60, 1895."

INDEX.

43.